Walt F.J. Goodridge, author of *A Clean Cell Never Dies*, *The Man Who Lived Forever* and publisher of *Fast & Grow Young*, and *The Power of Positive Eating* presents:

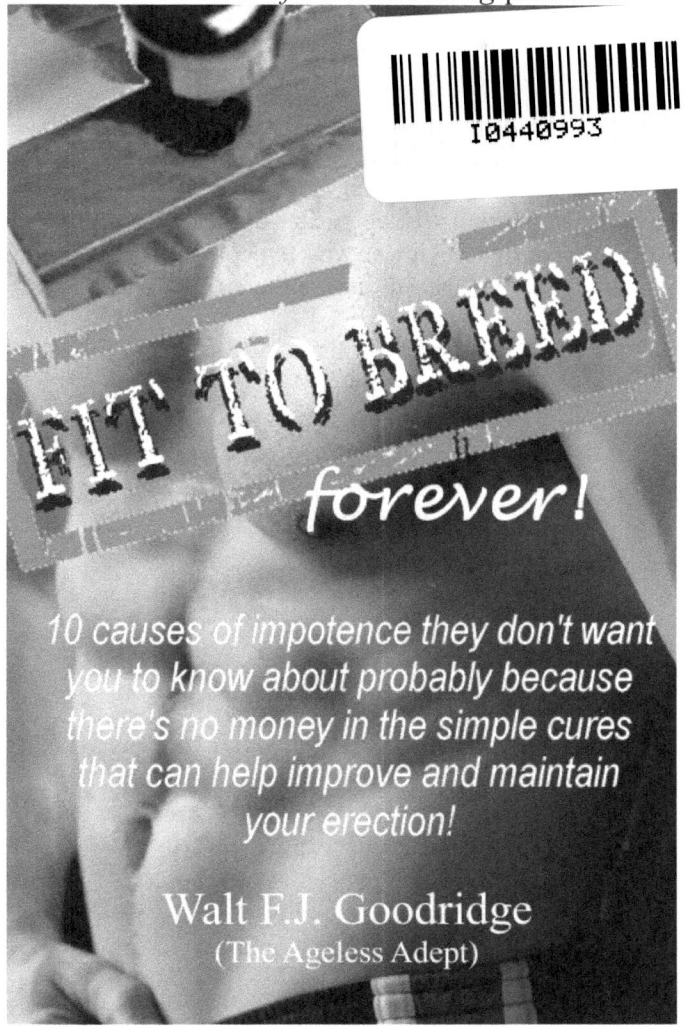

I0440993

FIT TO BREED

forever!

10 causes of impotence they don't want you to know about probably because there's no money in the simple cures that can help improve and maintain your erection!

Walt F.J. Goodridge
(The Ageless Adept)

Includes over 175 truths, principles, causes, cautions, motivation, myths and facts plus a proven protocol of practices, supplements, herbs, food, secret recipes and resources to help understand, improve, reverse, cure or avoid impotence...
... forever!

Fit to Breed...Forever!
The 10 Causes of Impotence They Don't Want You To Know
About Probably Because There's No Money in the Simple
Cures That Can Help Improve and Maintain Your Erection
(Volume 4 in the Ageless Adept™ Series)
© Walt F.J. Goodridge. All rights reserved.

Published by Walt F.J. Goodridge
dba a company called W
ISBN-13: 9781501099038 (AMAZ)
ISBN-13: 9798823125680 (B&N)
Cover Image: by CuraPhotography from 123RF.com

Visit a store called W

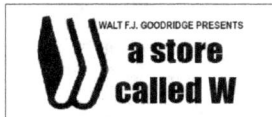

Books, apps, audio, video, merchandise,
courses, Walt's passion projects, freebies
and more from a company called W!
www.waltgoodridge.com/store

Distributed by
The Passion Profit Company
(646) 481-4238
www.PassionProfit.com
sales@passionprofit.com

Educational institutions, government agencies, libraries
and corporations are invited to inquire about quantity discounts.
Contact: sales@passionprofit.com

Printed in the United States of America

TABLE OF CONTENTS

The dedication ▲
This book is dedicated to my grandmother,
Isolene Rebecca Golding,
who taught me how to cook!
1907-1988

The acknowledgments ▲
Ken McRae, for putting me on the path
Thelma Goodridge, Christine St. Hilaire, Reina Joa,
Ernest & Kim Capers, Tony Cordoza, Andrew Morrison,
Aaron & Stacey Spencer-Willoughby, Kelly & Zelda Waters,
Diamond Davis, Nicole Drew, Carlton & Marian Gambrell,
Delxino & Deborah Wilson de Briano, Siew-Li Ng,
Chun Yu Wang, and Preeyaporn Promnoy Jompeang
for being part of the journey

My position ▲
"I am not here to convince, justify, defend or apologize
for my beliefs, choices or lifestyle. I'm not here for validation,
vindication or approval, nor to respond to personal attacks. I'm
here to share a philosophy & formula that work for me and that
work for others. In a world of seven billion people, if *one*
person can do a thing, then it *must* be possible for at least one
other person to do the same. It is against this backdrop that I
wrote this book."

❏ The necessary disclaimer▲❏

For legal reasons based on the prevailing societal paradigm, I must include the following:

The purpose of this guide is for me to provide my experiences and observations, and is intended for anyone who wants to learn more about my experiences staying young and fit to breed. I am not a doctor, and do not claim to be one.

The information in this guide is not intended to be a substitute for professional advice. It is only meant to complement, not replace any advice or information from a "health professional." You should not use this information to diagnose or treat health problems or disease without consulting a qualified "health care provider" with any questions or concerns you may have regarding your condition, or ways in which to use alternative medicine. I, the author of this book, disclaim any personal liability or loss caused or alleged to be caused, through application of the information in this guide.

As a result of each person's unique individual lifestyle, choices, history and path, each person's body has arrived at a unique place in its development, rejuvenation and/or deterioration and will, therefore, react differently, even to natural substances. As much as this guide contains merely suggestions of natural substances and natural practices, if you are currently on pharmaceutical medication of any kind, then your body's system is most likely compromised, and even natural foods could have an adverse effect on you.

Any strategy or protocol you implement must, therefore, be administered on an individual basis, and it would be wise to consult a holistic healing practitioner familiar with the contraindications of real food when combined with unnatural drugs and chemicals that may be present in your body.

The information contained herein is not intended to diagnose or prescribe treatment for any illness. Use the information contained herein as information only.

❏ Tip: How to use this manual ❏

(a) To get the most from this manual, never continue reading past a word or phrase you don't understand! It's been shown that the only reason people give up on a new project or course of study is that they encounter a word, phrase or concept for which they have no definition, or the wrong definition. If a word in this guide is new to you, please use a dictionary to find the most accurate definition. This is more important than people realize!

(b) Take the Fit to Breed™ Health Test! The latest version is at www.fittobreed.com. However, a shortened version is on page 115,

(c) Use the checkboxes! (❏) After you've read a particular idea/suggestion and understand how it relates to being fit to breed, check the box, initial it, date it, then proceed. Your initials represent a contract between your evolving self and your fit to breed ideal. (Hope you have the paperback version!) There's a second set of check boxes for a future reading.

(d) Investigate each item. This is not an encyclopedia. It's a guidebook. Think of it as a road map—a suggestion of an available route and destination with a checklist of sights and milestones along the way. It is up to you to take the time to explore each suggestion fully to really enjoy the journey!

(e) Read *Fit to Breed* twice—once for a general overview, and again to take action!

(f) Read *A Clean Cell Never Dies*, where you'll find detailed explanations of certain concepts, a review of principles

(g) Seek support. Share *Fit to Breed* with your partner(s). Hire a coach. Visit www.fittobreed.com and join the community!

🚫 = *products & protocols I have NOT tried personally.*

The Backdrop ▲

Who I am, why I wrote this,
and a few new ideas

1. ❑ Backdrop: Who I am ❑

My name is Walt F.J. Goodridge, author of a few books, including *Turn Your Passion Into Profit*, *Change the Game*, *Living True to Your Self*, *The Tao of Wow*, and *The Man Who Lived Forever*! Look me up!

2. ❑ Backdrop: Why I wrote this manual ❑

I wrote *this* manual because I discovered a secret. It is my belief, and thus my experience, and therefore my conclusion that it is not necessary for my sexual endurance and interest to decline as I spend more years on the planet, and that:

"Perfect health, long life and eternal youth are not the random genetic blessings of a chaotic or capricious universe, but natural birthrights that can be accessed through the mindful acceptance of simple truths, activated by the committed practice of proven activities, and sustained by advancement along a single known path. This is that path." -- **The Ageless Adept**, quoted in *The Man Who Lived Forever*

As a result of the things I've learned and currently

practice, my erections are stronger now than when in I was in college. I can "perform" for an average of two-four hours or more! I get compliments on my "taste." And, since I've disciplined myself to <u>not</u> ejaculate during every sexual session, not only can I bring porn star quality excitement, variety and creativity to my intimate encounters, but I maintain a high level of arousal that I can sublimate into my writing and other creative endeavors!

3. ❏ Backdrop: Who this manual is for ❏

This manual is ultimately for you if you're a man who'd like to honor, reclaim, retain, indulge and entertain his sexual interest, confidence, endurance, stamina and rigidity without the use of harmful drugs. It is also, of course, for your partner(s)... whether you want to actually "breed" or not!

4. ❏ Backdrop: What this manual contains ❏

I've had the good fortune (or perhaps it was a curse) of growing up Jamaican—an island culture in which male sexual prowess is celebrated in the lyrics of our songs, the connection between herbs and stamina is celebrated in the names of our beverages and tonics, where athletic dominance and courage (Usain, bobsledders) is par for the course, and from which Reggae—our gift to the world—drips not just of revolution, but sensuality as well. Reggae is as much "get up, stand up" as it is "take it off, lie down." It is an island where the satisfying experiences of the women who flock to our shores for hot tropical vacations—and I'm not talking weather—are legendary. Such a national reputation may have cast a heavy burden of expectation on this growing child, but it has imbued me with a certain respect for being "fit to breed!"

This manual, therefore, is my take on a phenomenon about which I as a man (and, perhaps as a Jamaican) have some insight. It grew out of my awareness that many men out there aren't pleasing their partners to the degree they (and definitely their women) would like to. (Don't ask me how I know!)

Okay, you've twisted my arm, so I'll tell you: In speaking with many *women* out there, I've discovered that the things *I* am able to do in the practice and pursuit of physical pleasure are apparently *not* the norm, and are not being duplicated by other men—for several reasons.

A few of those reasons include: lack of creativity, selfishness, laziness, or simply "plumbing malfunctions" a euphemism for erectile dysfunction—the inability of a man to achieve and sustain a viable erection during the act of sex.

Some of these malfunctions are mental and/or emotional in nature. Some of them are undoubtedly biological. As mentioned, some may be due to lack of creativity. While my inner porn star would love to offer interactive demonstrations on creative sexual techniques, I'll limit myself to addressing the physical, biological, mental and even cultural reasons for men's inability to achieve and maintain their erections.

This manual, therefore, contains over 200 *beliefs, truths, myths, principles, causes, supplements, herbs, foods, motivation, recipes and practices that have worked* for me, and that just might help others *understand, reverse, improve, cure and avoid impotence....and remain fit to breed forever!*

When I first started writing this guide, I was initially apprehensive about sharing this information under my real name. You see, over the years, I've established my brand with books on the music industry, starting passion-centered businesses, Internet marketing, and only recently, on achieving health. I suppose it was inevitable that, once into writing about health, I would eventually tackle the subject of sexual health. However, western society has erected (pun alert!) such taboo around it, that discussions of sexual enjoyment are often cause for secrecy and shame, and seen as an entirely separate area of expertise. After all, who takes sex advice from a business coach? (Don't kid yourself, we driven entrepreneurs have sex, too, and we might just be better at it!)

However, I made a decision a long time ago to live true to my self and my life's mission to *"share what I know, so that others may grow"* (pun alert!) in whatever ways and for whatever parts of the body that growth may apply!

With that said, you may discover things about me you may deem "TMI" (Too Much Information), and may find yourself covering your eyes and ears yelling *"Make him stop!"* However, it'll all be worth it, if better health is your objective.

So, let's throw caution to the wind, and in the famous and immortalized words of Salt n' Pepa, "Let's talk about sex!"

Walt F.J. Goodridge (aka The Ageless Adept)

"I share what I know,

so that others may grow!

p.s. To begin, there are two foundational ideas you'll need to accept and embrace to gain the most benefit from this book and others in this series:

5. ❑ Idea one: You are your own authority ❑

You don't need a PhD to understand your body, and you don't need anyone's permission to eat an apple. As eloquently spoken by author, Jerry Mander:

"[We must] make it easier for people to know about themselves, how they function, what a human being is, and how the human fits into the wider natural systems of the universe. This will make it possible for the human to recognize what is natural and real from what is artificial and contrived. People can achieve greater control of themselves, their needs, and their health, and find the answers they need on their own without the input of so-called experts and authorities from outside the self. Personal knowledge and experience is the best authority."

You can be your own authority, and *be* a "PhD" (pretty healthy dude) who wields a "PhD" (pretty hard, um, desire)!

(Find your status. Take the Fit to Breed Health Test at www.fittobreed.com)

6. ❑ Idea two: Everything you believe....is wrong❑

This house of cards we refer to as our society's current belief system is crumbling. The cloak of deception upon which that system was based is unraveling. Everything we've been told, believe and accept to be true about many aspects of reality is being challenged and exposed as simply false and wrong. Priests are being exposed as predators. Politicians are being exposed as agenda-driven individualists rather than selfless public servants. Everything we believe is "progress" is unsustainable and is propelling our planet towards extinction.

Everything you believe is "medicine" is often a set of untested drugs that unbalance the body's natural systems and cause more side effects than the illnesses they purport to cure.

Everything you believe is "food" are chemically-laden substances that are unusable by the body, clog the system, deprive and rob the body of nutrients and the ability to heal.

Everything you believe is "economic growth through capitalism" is actually a money-grab that only benefits a select few at the expense of everyone else.

Everything you believe is "justice" is a punitive, revenge-focused, violence-based system of thought and action that supports a prison industry designed to enrich its owners.

Everything you've been told are the random events of history might actually have been orchestrated.

Everything you believe to be "news" is sensationalized opinion and is, in many cases, completely contrived.

Everything you've been told to strive for in the pursuit of "success and freedom" actually leads to servitude and failure.

Everything you've been told, and thus believe is good, normal, necessary, desirable, ethical and moral are being revealed to be their exact opposites.

Everything you've been told and thus believe is evil sinful, impossible, absurd and abnormal might actually be good, ethical, plausible, logical, quite normal and, in fact, in your best interest to explore, once truth is revealed.

The list could go on and on. In our beliefs about science, democracy, religion, government, education, the causes of war, the reasons behind assassinations, the existence of life on other planets, the origin of mankind, sexuality and various other concepts, ideas institutions and world views—all are being subjected to the onslaught of new questions and analyses and then activism as people discover them to be other than what they've been led to believe is true.

Finally, everything you believe about the body and how to maintain it, as well as illness and how to avoid it...is wrong.

This may come as a surprise to you, but it's entirely possible that everything you believe to be true about food, medicine, health, illness and aging is nothing more than a set of subjective ideas put forth by people who really don't have a handle on truth, don't know what they're doing, or worse, don't have your best interests at heart—people who are playing by a faulty rule book or, worse, with no rule book at all.

Uninformed ideas, blind assumptions and outright lies underlie many of the food and drug commercials on television and radio. I'm sure you're familiar with many of these assumptions: that milk does a body good; that meat is real food for real people; that cancer can't be cured; that the common cold is inevitable; that allergies can only be relieved not ended; that hormone levels, hair growth and one's virility and vitality inevitably decrease at certain ages; and that drugs these companies are pushing heal and aren't, in fact, more dangerous than the ills they claim to cure, given the extensive list of (sometimes fatal) side effects warned of in the disclaimers.

The sales pitches for these products start with these assumptions as given and are never challenged. As a result, people buy into them (key word "buy'), and continue a vicious cycle perpetuating the very lifestyle that caused their ills.

Society has lost a vital road map and is devolving in a direction that serves to support the industries that profit from peddling the products--products allow people to believe they can maintain destructive lifestyles, while purchasing so-called "cures" that, in actuality, only temporarily relieve, mask or replace the symptoms of the illnesses the lifestyles cause.

If I believed, for example, that "milk does a body good," and then acted on that belief (by drinking lots of milk) in an effort to improve my health, I might find myself experiencing colds, mucous, allergies, weakened bones and cancer, and eventually become frustrated in my efforts to achieve health without ever knowing the real reason why: dairy products we've been told are beneficial, are, in fact poison to our systems!

For those pursuing a new paradigm of health, wellness, disease, aging and youth, what we need are:
- a lens of stable truths through which to see the world
- a new understanding of nature that encourages new questions
- a method of critical analysis to arrive at new answers
- a new set of possibilities and choices based on those answers
- a common sense philosophy on which to base your lifestyle practices, built upon a foundation of truths that never change.

In my own quest for those truths, I've met people who've cured lupus, sent their cancers into remission, gotten rid of allergies, eliminated colds, and live pain-free based on truths few are addressing or are ridiculed or suppressed. *(Excerpt from In Search of a Better Belief System. www.waltgoodridge.com)*

Over the next several chapters, I'm going to share with you truths that might help you understand the causes of impotence from an entirely different perspective, and then, how you can cure it in an equally truth-based way.

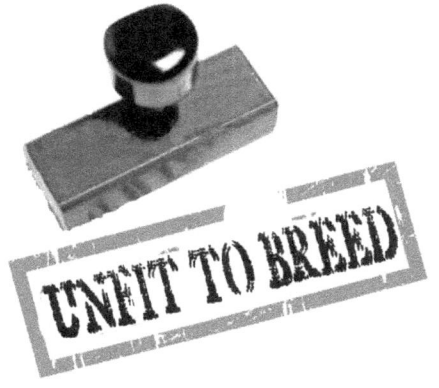

The Truth ▲

Necessary truths and principles
that will define our journey

7. ❑ Truth: The bottom line ❑

There is perhaps nothing more vital to a man's sense of well being and masculinity than his desire and ability to achieve and sustain an erection. Many products on the market seek to capitalize on this desire, and while some of these products are perceived as effective in the short-term, none will ever be completely effective or safe in actually curing impotence. I can say this with absolute certainty because all these so-called remedies or cures are missing the point entirely on what *really* causes impotence, and thus, how to actually reverse it.

If you are among the millions of men who suffer from some form of erectile dysfunction, lowered libido, depressed sex drive or impotence, or even if you're okay but concerned about the future, I'll share with you a simple truth:

If you are impotent, it is because Nature has classified you as "UNFIT TO BREED."
Let me repeat a little "louder:"

"You are impotent because Nature has classified you "UN-FIT to breed!"

Furthermore, until you are *re-classified* as "FIT to Breed," your impotence will continue and worsen. Now before you get too depressed by that sobering bit of news, let me share with you the *good* news. The good news is that yes, you *can* actually change your classification!

And, while you may be much more interested in simply getting to that reclassification strategy, if you can really understand your situation in the unique way I'm about to share with you, you will understand why the "cure" I recommend is the only one that can ever truly be effective in the long term.

Before I explain how to get reclassified, let's understand how and why the classification occurs in the first place. To do that, we need to understand seven specific truths that govern everything in the universe, and then we need to learn a few specific principles based on those truths and how they apply to matters of health and wellness, and specifically to impotence.

The 7 Truths of Reality

These 7 Truths are known worldwide by mystics, philosophers, sages and seekers of all stripes, and shared by adepts of all spiritual paths. They are the basic, essential truths that *should* be taught in every school, but for reasons that belong in a different type of manual, they are often hidden from the masses. (Search online in the public domain for "Kybalion.")

8. ❑ Truth 1: The Truth of Mind ❑

The first truth, the *Truth of Mind*, holds that all reality starts first as thought and belief. To achieve any desired end, therefore, you must first make yourself believe in the reality of what you wish to achieve. As it relates to this discussion, you must first believe it is possible and inevitable that you will eventually become fit to breed.

9. ❑ Truth 2: The Truth of Correspondence ❑

Second is the *Truth of Correspondence* that states 'as above, so below.' What is truth above must be truth below. Stated still in another way, if a principle is true in matters of spirit, then it must be true in matters of flesh, otherwise it is not truth. If something claims to be truth but has contradictions, conditions, catches (or a whole bunch of side effects), then it is most likely either a religion or an advertisement for a prescription drug! Ouch!

The bases of the Fit to Breed philosophy and formula are observable and provable in other areas of life.

10. ❑ Truth 3: The Truth of Motion ❑

Third is the *Truth of Motion* that states that everything in the universe is in a state of motion. Everything vibrates. Every object, every action, every thought and every state of being is merely energy in a unique state of vibration and motion.

In other words, nothing is fixed or motionless or unchangeable—good to know when seeking to be fit to breed.

11. ❑ Truth 4: The Truth of Duality ❑

Fourth is the *Truth of Duality* that states that everything is one thing. Extremes of anything are just degrees of that same thing. There is always *only* one thing. In other words, *"...opposites are identical in nature, but different in degree."* For example, heat and cold are really the same thing (temperature) differing only in degree. So too are black and white, love and hate, east and west. Similarly, health and illness are the same thing differing only in degree. In any effort to change a thing, there must be the recognition that the path of change goes from one pole to the other. The path from illness to health (eg. from impotence to being fit to breed), therefore, can be conceptualized as just such a direct path.

12. ❑ Truth 5: The Truth of Rhythm ❑

Fifth is the *Truth of Rhythm* that states that all things rise and fall. There is always action and reaction, back and forth, high tide and low tide, inflow and outflow in all things that affect the ways and worlds of men, including health.

13. ❑ Truth 6: The Truth of Cause and Effect ❑

Sixth is the *Truth of Cause and Effect* that states nothing is random. Everything you experience is the direct result of some cause. As it relates to health, you are always "at cause" for your health. Your thoughts are first cause, your actions are the means, and the conditions of your body are the effects.

It may *seem* like a mystery why sometimes "it" works and sometimes it doesn't. However, health is not a mystery, and illness is not random. Both proceed by the law of cause and effect. You get each to the degree you create it.

14. ❑ Truth 7: The Truth of Gender ❑

Seventh is the *Truth of Gender* that states there is masculine and feminine in all things. Whenever anything is created, whether on a physical, mental or spiritual plane, the principles of father/mother, God/Nature, seed/womb are always in operation. Creation, generation, regeneration and the secret to creating youthfulness, all rely on this truth.

These truths comprise the totality of every phenomenon we know to exist and those we don't. Everything in the universe is based on these simple, stable truths. If the universe were not based on reliable, predictable truths, everything would collapse.

These truths are vital to our discussion of impotence, and for our understanding of cure. Two in particular, the Truth of Duality (that everything is one thing and therefore reversible), and the Truth of Cause and Effect (that nothing is random), are particularly important. Keep them in mind.

The Principles

The following principles are based on the 7 truths just discussed. It is essential you understand and accept the first principle for the ones that follow to make sense.

15. ❑ Principle: Nature is foolproof ❑

Nature, as a whole thing, survives via the survival of its individual components—plants, animals, oceans, ecosystems etc. The activities of survival are simple enough so that one does *not* need higher degrees to grasp or execute them: Predators seek prey. Animals mate by instinct. Seeds grow by design. Bees pollinate flowers. Animals seek brightly colored fruit. Everything proceeds seamlessly in ways that are foolproof (i.e. even a fool couldn't screw them up!)

In *The Man Who Lived Forever*, the adept questions the seeker about nature and God*:

"Seeker, if you were God, perfect, wise and omnipotent —would you create a world and a system of survival that required PhDs to master? Or would you make it foolproof, so that even the least of your creations could negotiate it?

"I guess I'd make it simple," I replied.

"And the truth is, Seeker, it is simple. God is not complicated. Complex, vast and infinite, perhaps, but not complicated. Nature is a simple, closed, self-contained system coded for survival. In other words, everything Nature needs for its own survival is already built right in. It's a 'batteries included' universe, if you will."

*Becoming fit to breed does not require belief in a deity. Universal order is observable regardless of that part of your belief system.

16. ❏ Principle: Nature is coded for survival ❏

Yes, Nature is coded for survival. Its prime directive is the continuation of itself. Furthermore, the human body—your body—as one of the component parts of Nature, is an *agent* of Nature's survival. It has also been designed and coded to support Nature's survival. Your sex drive, desire and ability to breed support the survival of the species to which you belong. Breeding is how any organism and thus how any species survives and perpetuates itself.

It is a prime directive of everything on the planet that, right after basic survival, breeding comes next on the list as the thing we are compelled to do. Your libido, your sex drive and your interest in sex, are all part of your coding that supports nature's survival. Organisms that possess the best genes to perpetuate the species are allowed to breed.

Now, since it's an established fact that men can produce viable sperm well into their later years, then the common explanation of "you're getting old" cannot possibly be the reason your libido, sex drive and ability to maintain an erection don't also sustain themselves well into later years. I suggest that if your sperm is viable, but your "plumbing" doesn't work, it's not because the body is incapable of it. It is because Nature has assessed your worthiness and does not want you to breed!

Nature, through your body's built-in coding, lessens your sex drive to keep you from spreading 'weak' seed that will result in offspring that stand less chance of survival and more chance of dooming the species.

Think about it. As far as Nature is concerned, the purpose of sex is to create healthy offspring to continue the species. Therefore, any trait or condition that reduces the potential health and survivability of the resulting offspring will be classified as 'undesirable,' and any organism exhibiting those traits will be classified as unfit to breed.

Furthermore, Nature's *response* to anything that attempts to subvert that directive will also be unavoidable. In other words, if you try to override Nature's prime directive by using drugs to "fool" nature, or to find a "loophole" in the classification decision, Nature will take further steps to punish the violation. It's now being shown that Viagra causes vision deterioration. That makes sense. Nature—in response to your attempts to circumvent its classification—takes more extreme measures to further prevent you from breeding. If you try to circumvent the natural lowering of your sex drive, Nature takes remedial action and deprives you of sight—a major hindrance to arousal, especially for the male of the species. See how it works? Nature's directive will not be denied.

17. ❑ Principle: The body is coded to heal ❑

As an individual unit of nature, your body is coded for healing, reversal, regeneration, renewal and rejuvenation. Cuts heal. Broken bones mend. Fevers kill germs. Yes, provided with the raw materials it needs, and left to its own intelligence, the body is designed to do what it needs to in order to heal, survive, and thrive. Everything you currently define as illness is actually healing taking place. Diarrhea, colds, coughs are all efforts by your body to cleanse and heal itself.

We're even told by experts that the body's organs renew themselves regularly, and that the entire body is completely renewed every seven years. You might ask, "*If the body is coded to heal, why am I and everyone I know deteriorating, and why am I impotent?*" As your own authority, you'll answer that question yourself by the time you finish this manual.

First, however, let's explore how an individual body actually becomes *un-fit* to breed in the first place.

18. ❑ Principle: There is only one illness ❑

Arnold Ehret, Charlotte Gerson and other healers have all shown and stated in their own ways that there is only one illness. (Remember, everything is one thing.) Un-reversed, this one illness starts to manifest in different parts of the body. However, it is a single issue that is at cause. Ehret refers to it as constipation. Gerson refers to it as toxicity. I call it "blockage."

Blockage means (a) there is something *inside* the body that is being blocked from coming out, or (b) something *outside* the body that is being blocked from coming in. There is something that was ingested or absorbed that stayed in. Or something missing that must be assimilated. Illness is *always* either an accumulation or a void of some kind.

Blockage (or constipation, or toxicity) occurs when things are introduced into the body that are not in harmony with our coding. We eat processed, refined, artificially flavored, colored, pasteurized, homogenized, fried, filtered and altered food, that is simply not natural. The body, which was never designed to handle these unnatural substances, suffers from accumulations and deposits and gets clogged. These clogs result in increased toxicity. The toxicity gets chronic (persisting for a long time), and deterioration results. The body's natural code is further suppressed, and more disease results.

Conversely, the flip side of blockage is depletion. We eat depleted foods and never adequately replenish the depletion of vitamins, minerals etc. the body requires for optimal function and to execute its healing code. The mystery is not why we get sick. The real mystery is how we stay alive given all the damage and depletion to which we subject ourselves.

19. ❑ Principle: There is only one cure ❑

If there is only one illness, it stands to reason there is only one cure. Since blockage is what we're dealing with, the cure must be something that creates the opposite of blockage. The opposite of blockage is FLOW.

The Truth of Rhythm says where there is 'inflow' there must be 'outflow.' So if blockage (the illness) implies a blockage of intake and output, then flow (the cure) must imply a flow in as well as a flow out. Eating is inflow. Elimination is outflow. The two working together form the basis of health.

As flow improves, health results. As flow decreases and becomes blockage, disease and illness result. The cure for blockage, and thus the cure for all illness is flow.

According to the Truth of Rhythm, every "in" must have an "out." For every assimilation, there must be a corresponding elimination. The simple reason why many people in this society are ill is because they never give their bodies the time or the means to eliminate.

Every illness that is the result of accumulation can be cured by release. Similarly, every illness that is the result of depletion can be cured by replenishment. Ninety percent of all blockage can be cured simply by allowing the body the time and raw materials it needs to return to a state of flow.

20. ❑ Principle: A clean cell never dies ❑

Excerpt: "Back in the 1920s, Nobel Prize laureate Dr. Alexis Carrel began his famous experiment in which he proved that living cells could be kept alive indefinitely by simply controlling the nutrients and waste removal in the surrounding solution. After 28 years, the original chicken liver cells were still alive in the Petri dish, and Dr. Carrel's point was proven. There are two main requirements for cells to stay alive: proper nutrients, and removal of wastes. With a blocked colon, all the body's cells suffer. Autointoxication poisons the entire body, all its tissues, and all its organs. This can be the cause of practically any disease, especially those conditions listed in the pathology books as "cause unknown." "--[from *The Doctor Within*]

21. ❏ Principle: Impotence is a bad habit ❏

Now, let's apply what we've just learned to the issue of impotence. This illness called impotence is nothing more than the specific manifestation of a chronic condition that has been developing as a result of certain practices over the years.

Imagine that your health at any single moment in time is represented by a single point along a line. Let's say this line has 26 points each represented by the letters of the alphabet. Your health journey, therefore, would look something like this:

```
A  B  C  D  E  F  G  H  I  J  K  L...
------------------------------->
```

Further, let's say the letter "I" represents the symptoms of impotence.

As you go through life living that habitual lifestyle, accumulations and depletions occur, the flow gets blocked, and you begin deteriorating and progressing along this line—moving further and further to the right. Perhaps at age 30 you start experiencing some "A" symptoms, then a few months or years later, some "B" symptoms. By the time you start noticing full blown "I" (impotence) symptoms that don't improve on their own, you may already be at point J, K or L on the path. In other words, starting many years ago, you got into the bad habit of making yourself impotent, and now it is starting to manifest!

Furthermore, this systemic deterioration will usually

have numerous other manifestations beyond just your "I" symptoms. Any or all of those additional symptoms could give Nature reason enough to revoke your "procreation pass." In other words, by the time you get to "I" and beyond, there could be many conditions affecting not only the strength and vitality of your sperm and your reproductive machinery, but your overall health as well.

For instance, by the time you get to "I" and beyond, you may have accumulated heavy metals in your organs or blood.

You may have accumulated worms and other parasites in your organs, blood or system.

You may have the accumulated effects of an overly acidic system, a condition that causes free-radical damage and ultimately devolves into cancer.

You may be depleted in several critical nutrients, enzymes, vitamins and minerals.

You may have a depleted digestive, endocrine, nervous, lymph or other vital system.

We could go on.

The point is—as you can see—true cure cannot simply be about addressing your "I" symptoms. We've got to look at the bigger picture. The only way to cure your impotence is to somehow get back to point "H" which is where you were, say at age 30 just before your "I" symptoms started to appear, and continue to points prior. Our objective is to halt the decline, and reverse the overall trend and the direction of your health path.

22. ❑ Principle: Everything is reversible ❑

Yes, it's like going back in time. But as we first learned in *Yesterday's You*, everything is reversible. If you arrived at point "I" by eating French fries every day, then to start reversing the trend, it is simply necessary to stop eating French fries, *and* to take some remedial action as well. There is no way around it. Your present condition is the direct result of actions you have taken—things done as well as things *not* done—so reversing these actions and non-actions is the *only* way to truly reverse your condition! Please read that statement again and embrace it. It holds the key to your success becoming fit to breed.

By addressing the release of accumulation and the replenishment of depletion that true health requires, and allowing your body the time it needs to naturally heal itself, you will be strengthening your immune system, correcting imbalances, ridding yourself of parasites, reducing your body's level of toxicity, acidity, and as a result you will stop and reverse the body's deterioration. Then, and only then will Nature re-open your case and consider reclassifying you, and upgrading your status to fit to breed.

I know that this may seem like a tall order, but remember: the body is naturally coded to heal. All *you* have to do is simply support it naturally, and allow it the time and environment to do what it is already coded to do.

Now, this "cure" won't be for everybody. Few people in our modern, "magic dust," "overnight fix" society, truly possess the commitment to change their habits. Therefore, they opt for what they believe is a quick remedy. Again, this is a matter of personal choice. You are free to make any choice at all. Just remember, however, according to the Truth of Cause and Effect, that every choice has consequences.

23. ❑ Truth: Drugs can't solve this ❑

Opting for the quick fix means you'll be addressing the *symptoms* of what is likely a deeper, more serious condition, by putting substances in your body that are unnatural. When those unnatural substances accumulate as well, you'll be setting your self up for your overall health to worsen in ways you never imagined. I remind you again of the many side effects of all the unnatural substances the medical establishment refers to as medicine. Keep in mind:

1. Addressing only the symptom means that the root cause of your impotence remains unaddressed and will lead to other complications.

2. Taking these untested pills and remedies will cause other accumulation or depletion in the body that will cause other bodily systems to swing out of balance.

3. Every UN-natural remedy has side effects that, while they may be acceptable to you in light of the payoff (a functioning plumbing system), are nevertheless constantly furthering the body's deterioration, and will result in the ultimate ineffectiveness of the original "cure." (Remember, Viagra™ and the "blindness" side effect. That's sheer insanity, if you really think about it! What's the point of having an erection if you can't visually enjoy the beauty of your partner's reaction and the sight of their pleasure?)

So, as tedious as this Fit to Breed cure may seem at first, it is the only viable solution to what ails you.

Remember: There's nothing man can develop or devise

that can be an improvement over nature in its original state.

The reason the established medical industry won't (can't) ever successfully create a real, side-effect-free, biologically safe, environmentally respectful cure for impotence is that impotence, like any other affliction is simply a symptom of a gradual deterioration of the body along a path. Reversing that path is the only cure.

Everything else that you can buy (Viagra™, et.al) avoids the causes and provides a quick fix that's not really a fix at all. It is avoidance. It is compromise. It is delusion.

However, there is a better solution. There are things you can do, and steps you can take to encourage the flow and thus the health of your compromised, unfit system. As you do, you'll discover some amazing things about the incredible simplicity of the human body, and the grand design it is a part of. Before we get to the healing protocol for reversing toxicity and depletion as the cause of impotence, let's summarize some of the other lesser-known reasons for impotence.

The Causes ▲

A short list of what may be causing
your plumbing malfunction.

24. ❑ Cause one: You're unfit to breed ❑

Some impotence is caused by
bodily toxicity and depletion
Nature has re-classified you as UNFIT to breed

As discussed, some impotence is caused by bodily toxicity and depletion. There are *substances* (sugar, salt, caffeine, nicotine, alcohol, dairy, meat, fat), as well as *environments* (air conditioning, fluorescent lights, electromagnetic fields, microwaves, pollution), *lifestyles* (inactivity, lack of sunlight, stress, tension, even 9-to-5 employment), and *organisms* (parasites, bacteria, viruses) that have caused imbalance, deterioration, depletion and toxicity in your body, making you such a poor candidate to perpetuate the species, that Nature had to reclassify you as "UNFIT to Breed."

Although the most likely, it is just one possible cause. Let's explore some additional mental, emotional, societal, genetic and even cultural factors:

25. ❑ Cause two: It's Just a "First time failure" ❑

I believe that some impotence
is caused by "The Familiar First Time Failure"
In other words, "I hardly know you!"

It's actually been shown that men are more turned on by familiarity, and that women are more turned on by strangers. In other words, a woman will be more sexually excited by the prospect of being with a *stranger*, while a man will be more sexually excited by the prospect of being with someone who's more personally known and more *familiar* to him. If that's true, it means that, despite the prevailing stereotype—that men are perpetually horny and ever-ready to consummate—the reality may be that a man's interest, attraction and hence, sexual arousal and performance grow over time as he becomes more familiar with his partner.

This could certainly explain what I refer to as the "First Time Failure," an anecdotally prevalent situation in which a man simply cannot achieve an erection, or experiences premature ejaculation just moments into (sometimes even before) actual penetration with a new partner. We guys write it off as the consequence of the heightened excitement of "the first time," or as "performance anxiety," or as getting accustomed to the newness of our partner. The fact may be that we're simply not turned on enough because it takes a little time. However, many men view this situation as an indication of impotence, and may then doom themselves by turning their fears and anxiety into self-fulfilling prophecies.

From my own experience, it has taken me sometimes two or three encounters before I've built up enough familiarity, comfort, history and the feeling of anticipation of being with my lover before things to start to work as they eventually do.

26. ❑ Cause three: Incompatible DNA ❑

I believe that some impotence
is caused by incompatible DNA
In other words, the two of you
are simply not meant to breed
Pheromones may be to blame!

I once met a young lady. We hit it off well. She was attractive. She was vegetarian, and had a nice personality. When we finally got together inside my apartment, however, things didn't quite seem to work, and I had a "plumbing malfunction!" Not a problem, I thought to myself. Must be the "First Time Failure." It'll be better next time!

Now, the second night we got together was outdoors on the beach. We started our play date, and things appeared to be working fine. However, once we got back to my apartment, guess what? Plumbing malfunction again! Darn! I sensed a pattern.

The third night we got together was outdoors again. It was our final night together as she was returning to her homeland that evening. Things went great and we had a great time....all outdoors! But, the question haunts me to this day. Why didn't things work when we were indoors? Was it performance anxiety? Or was it something else? After much analysis, I've come to my own conclusion.

A pheromone is a chemical an animal produces that changes the behavior of another animal of the same species. Pheromones are naturally occurring, odorless substances the fertile body excretes externally, conveying an airborne signal that provides information to, and triggers responses from the opposite sex of the same species. And while some medical literature reject the existence of pheromones in humans, I personally have no reason to believe that Nature's intelligence is not also at work in the human species. ("As above, so below.")

It's been shown that the sense of smell and the effect of pheromones are critical components of one's sexual arousal and thus, sexual compatibility. I now believe that when my date and I were outdoors in the cool summer breeze, things were fine. However, being in close quarters with her allowed the pheromones to take effect and caused my plumbing malfunction. I believe, in other words, that Nature had deemed our DNA to be incompatible, but the manifestation of that fact didn't become apparent until we were indoors together with no breezes blowing to "dilute" the pheromones. I call it my *indoor* plumbing malfunction! Strange.

Consequently, I believe some "impotence" is simply nature's warning not to breed! Eventually, however, familiarity, or pent-up desire, or some other factor gets things working fine, and people disregard this warning of basic incompatibility. However, such basic chemical incompatibility may rear its head again some time later and result in impotence.

Has this ever happened to you??? Email me and/or share at comments@fittobreed.com!

27. ❑ Cause four: She's just not your type ❑

I believe that some impotence is caused
by dating lovers who simply aren't your type

For many men in our society, sex partners are so difficult to come by, that many men are simply glad when they find someone at all, and feel they don't have the luxury of *choosing* their "type." Many people have particular preferences of height, weight, ethnic background, shoe size, facial features, etc., but end up settling for whomever is available and willing.

It's no wonder, then, that such couplings end up being unfulfilling and ultimately lose their initial spark and chemistry —if indeed there was any there to begin with.

You're not being "shallow" by acknowledging, honoring and acting on the fact that you're wired to be turned on by certain attributes more so than by others. That's what dating and mating is all about. Nature designed it that way. Don't fight it.

Yes, I believe that a lot of impotence is caused by couples operating in a paradigm of desperation and settling for whomever's available, rather than choosing one's type!

28. ❑ Cause five: Incompatible DOMS & subs ❑

I believe that some impotence
is caused by incompatible
dominance & submission wiring

This cause is somewhat related to the previous one. Beyond the visual, physical attributes that attract us to each other, I've discovered there are some less visible, but probably even more important wiring that makes us ultimately compatible or not. I'm referring now to the concepts of "dominance" and "submission."

If you are to gain a better handle on how you're wired, understand what attracts you, honor your libido, heighten your sexual pleasure and satisfaction, it will be necessary to know where you fall in the range of being a "Dom" or being a "sub."

Now, dominance and submission in this context has nothing to do with your education, economic status or even your gender. It has nothing to do with societal subjugation of one gender over another. In fact, some women are "DOMS" and some men are "subs." However, all other things being equal, if you are a heterosexual male who falls somewhere in the normal distribution of the bell curve of dominance, you will likely be attracted to women who fall somewhere in the normal distribution of the bell curve of submission. That's just how Nature has it wired.

The challenge is that in our society, those two words have been co-opted and bastardized so that many people—and women in particular—hear them quite negatively.

In the gay community, the somewhat related terms "top" and "bottom" are used in awareness that there are certain recognizable roles/wiring in sexual interaction. Within the hetero community, however, society has pit men and women in competition with each other and brainwashed people into thinking that there is a power struggle for "dominance" that one or the other must "win" in order to be "equal."

Not all societies are thus afflicted. Other societies recognize inherent gender differences and without belittling each other, and without assuming a combative posture, retain a comfort and acceptance of the reality that men are generally wired one way, and women are generally wired in another.

Men and women are NOT the same. As I always say, *if we're both going to be the same in this relationship, then one of us is unnecessary!*

We can be equal in our "differentness."

Regardless of what transpires in the work-a-day world, some people are wired and thus more comfortable in their sexual identities, roles and interactions being more dominant, while others are wired and thus more comfortable, desirous and thus more aroused and more satisfied being more submissive.

My point is: If you're NOT aware if you're a DOM or a sub in your sexual identity and nature, then find some tests online. Knowing this critical fact about yourself can be the most liberating thing you can discover. It will help you be more comfortable with who you are. It will help you be clearer about who you should be choosing as your partners.

For, try as you might, if you are a man seeking to be a dominant man, but finding yourself with similarly dominant women, then no matter how hard you try, you'll simply never feel like a man. And, in match-ups like this, it's no wonder the plumbing doesn't work!

For more on this topic, check out *"Masculinity Version 2.0" A man's guide for setting standards, living and loving true to your self, getting and satisfying the women you want...all without EVER compromising your masculinity* at http://www.masculinity2.com

29. ❑ Cause six: Being in the wrong society ❑
I believe that some impotence
is caused by being in the wrong society
You might be happier abroad!

If you are feeling unfulfilled in your quest for romance and find yourself impotent, part of the reason may actually be the pond in which you're fishing. It's entirely possible—given the way our society has developed (i.e. the adversarial nature of male-female relationships, the de-feminization of women, and de-masculization of men)—that you are, quite bluntly, living in the "wrong" society!

As you evolve as a man—or simply as a person, for that matter—you may find there are things about a specific society that become more appealing. Likewise, there may be things about a specific society that become *less* appealing. Remember, these imaginary lines painted across the earth that separate us in terms of countries are all an arbitrary construct that you can choose not to let restrict your options.

"Imagine there's no countries....
it's easy if you try...."
--John Lennon

For various reasons including different climate, culture, gender roles, standards of living, etc., you might find yourself more satisfied, more fulfilled and may find others who elicit a different emotional as well as physical response in you.

I invite you to check out a website called "Happier Abroad" (www.happierabroad.com), filled with stories of men who've found what they've been looking for in other societies and cultures. It's a pretty interesting site!

"Sure, Walt, but things were working here in my homeland when I was younger! If I was in the wrong society, it wouldn't have worked then, right?"

Valid point, but societies do change over time. Not only that, men—meaning YOU—may change over time, too. And, as I've alluded to before, the honeymoon of excitement that comes with your first youthful explorations and adventures into sex can mask many situations that become more evident as the blush fades and as you mature. And, don't forget that impotence develops over time due to chronic bad habits!

Warning: If your impotence is, in fact, physiological, make sure you address it before you go traipsing around the world looking for love in all the wrong places. If you're unfit to breed in your home country, you'll be unfit to breed everywhere else. At the same time, I'm sure many men will find at least partial explanations for their puzzling plumbing malfunctions once they seek their bliss abroad!

30. ❏ Cause seven: Lack of fulfillment ❏

I believe that some impotence
is caused by lack of overall fulfillment
Is this all there is? I'm just not feelin' it anymore!

As the years progress, what may actually be changing is not your plumbing, but your purpose and your passions; in other words, your sense of fulfillment. *Passion* in this context refers to those hobbies or interests that inspire you.

As you play all the roles and do all the things society requires of you, you may simply not feel like a man or the success you'd like to be. Sometimes, that sense of disillusionment becomes more pronounced as we mature and we start to realize that sexual adventurism is not the "be all and end all" of our definition of self, and that there is a greater purpose and unexplored passions that we've been neglecting.

At that juncture in our development, the very act of sex may become a reminder of our lack of fulfillment—and who can get excited about that? Who can get excited when it becomes increasingly more apparent that the outcomes, validation and gender reinforcement we've been led to associate with sex repeatedly fall short of our expectations as well as our inner needs? Yes, sometimes, lack of overall fulfillment in life manifests as impotence.

31. ❏ Cause eight: Not the right team ❏

I believe that some impotence
is caused by unacknowledged
sexual orientation

There are many men who, due to societal, family or religious pressure, find themselves forced to adopt a heterosexual lifestyle and play for the straight team, even though they've been wired for homosexuality.

I believe that some impotence can be the result of not being true to one's self in terms of one's sexual orientation.

32. ❏ Cause nine: Being tone deaf ❏

I believe that some impotence
is caused by people
operating at lower tone levels

According to one theory, emotions follow a hierarchy. This hierarchy is called the Tone Scale. As you move up the tone scale, life improves. As you move down the scale, life gets worse. Here are a few milestones on the tone scale and numeric values associated with each:

enthusiasm 4.0

cheerfulness 3.0

contentment 2.8

boredom 2.5

anger 1.5

fear 1.0

grief 0.5

apathy 0.05

According to the theory, most people in society are operating at 2.5 and below—between apathy and boredom. More significantly, each level of emotional operation also carries a corresponding susceptibility to illness:

At 3.0, the individual is *"resistant to infection and disease"* and has *"few psychosomatic ills"* with an *"interest in procreation."*

At 2.5, the individual is *"occasionally ill, and susceptible to the usual diseases"* with a *"disinterest in procreation"*

At 2.0, the individual has *"severe sporadic illnesses,"* and exhibits a *"disgust and revulsion with sex."*

At 1.5, the individual has *"depository illnesses (like arthritis),"* has a lot of anger, and "*uses sex as punishment via rape.*"

You can see that if a man is operating around 2.5, with a disinterest in procreation, that, by definition, impotence is the natural result. The goal, therefore, is to raise one's level of emotional operation whether through personal development, therapy, or other means in order to function at a higher tone!

33. ❏ Cause ten: Soul-specific sublimation ❏
*I believe that some impotence
is caused by a higher consciousness
seeking expression in our lives*

Have you, or anyone you know ever been referred to as an "old soul?" It's a common expression, used to identify a person (often a child) whose personality, perspective, attitudes, interests, knowledge, abilities, demeanor, visage and/or aura seem to suggest he's been here (on this planet) before.

It stands to reason that if there are "old" souls, there must also be "young" souls, and souls of every "age" in between. Well—according to philosophers, mystics, seers and sages who, for centuries have observed, experienced or channeled information about this concept—there are!

The soul age concept is based on the idea that our immortal souls have had many different experiences on this plane of existence, and that some of us souls—in the ongoing adventure to experience all there is—have been here many times, in different identities, while other souls have had fewer "repeats" or are new to the earth school. Whatever your views on reincarnation, the idea that people are born with varying levels of spiritual development and maturity is indisputable.

The concept holds that there are five states—or ages—of soul development: *Infant, Baby, Young, Mature* and *Old*; each with its own set of challenges, motivations and aspirations:

Infant Souls are driven by fear, and challenged with basic survival. There is little feeling for ethics or personal morality. Love and sexuality are experienced on the level of lust.

Baby Souls are more comfortable in the world, less fear-driven, but require structure in order to feel comfortable. They want direction and seek out higher authorities to set clear rules for them. Traditions, rituals, and law and order provide them a welcomed sense of security.

Young Souls having mastered the issues of survival, discipline and order, are now looking to see how powerful they can become in the world. Ambition, status, power, wealth, and the ability to get what one wants out of life are the driving forces of the Young Soul.

Mature Souls tend to focus less on the outer world and the material, and more on the inner world as well as relationship issues. The questions "Who am I?" and "Why am I here?" are asked with frequency in these lives. Emotions open up, and boundaries between people break down. Non-traditional religions, meditation, and metaphysics start to look interesting.

Old Souls have detached from the emotional intensities of the Mature Soul period and are more objective about the ups and downs of life. According to The Michael Teachings (See www.michaelteachings.com):

"Even sex is not highly prized by the Old soul. He is

usually competent therein, but his lack of interest for it, and the lack of passion in it, can be disconcerting to younger souls who still prize sex highly. Old souls are often androgynous (having balanced masculine and feminine characteristics), and occasionally bisexuality is a part of their lifestyle. Gender identification is often weak in this Age because of subconscious contact with the whole psyche, which includes masculine and feminine characteristics. What the Old soul seeks in romantic relationships is a "soul mate" — someone to whom he relates on a soul level. This might be someone else with whom he has spent many lifetimes, or another soul in his own Entity."

Can you relate? If so, perhaps something more profound is at the root of your so-called impotence. The old, enlightened soul operates less from lower carnal chakras (energy centers), and more from higher realms of thought and action.

The process by which sexual energy is used for "higher' more creative purposes is called sublimation. As a writer, if I were to indulge all of my sexual urges, I likely would not have written the 20-plus books and hundreds of articles I have. When compared to the prevailing stereotype of maleness, it probably appears my sexual interest is low. In fact, it's quite the opposite. However, I simply cannot "get it up" for just any woman! I suggest to you that if your desire for sex is similar, that you consider the possibility there is some old soul-specific sublimation you are here to do that demands your attention!

34. ❏ Bonus Cause: Daddy Depressant? ❏

While a correlation has been known to exist in animals, a study in 2011 showed a drop in testosterone in men once those men became fathers with the role of caregiver! Nature's directive? Perhaps, but don't worry, it wasn't a connection to impotence, merely a small decrease in testosterone!

The Caveats ▲

caveat: n. a warning or proviso of specific stipulations,
conditions or limitations

35. ❑ Caveat: not by pill but by path ❑

Before we explore the cures for impotence, I need to
share what is perhaps the most important concept of all. As you
review the following suggested strategies and substances, your
goal should be to start yourself moving on a *path* during which
time you implement as many of these strategies and incorporate
as many of them as possible into your daily, weekly, monthly
and annual lifestyle, behavior, cooking and eating in order to
create and sustain lasting change in your situation.

These cures are NOT a list within which to find one or
two quick "fixes" that work for you while you continue to
engage in a destructive lifestyle. They should be seen as the
elements of an overall *improved* lifestyle you should strive to
adopt. This may require that you reprogram yourself from the
"pill as cure" mindset that our society promotes.

I cannot stress this enough. True and lasting cure is
never something that comes from a pill. It is something that
comes as the effect of a process—a path. You must commit
yourself to the path if you are ever to achieve the designation of
being fit to breed…forever!

36. ❏ Caveat: Your mileage may vary ❏

It was a few years after college that a Muslim friend questioned me about my consumption of pork. He asked questions about my dietary choices, what was in my food, and how those foods were affecting my health. Quite honestly, I was clueless, and it bothered me that I didn't have the answers to those simple questions. So, on my own, I started immersing myself in information about diet and vegetarianism. Some of the first books I read were *How to Eat to Live, Diet for a New America, Why Do Vegetarians Eat Like That*, and *Back to Eden*.

Armed with this information, and on my own authority, I stopped eating meat. One day I was an omnivore, the next day I was vegetarian. No more beef, pork, chicken or shellfish. No more eggs, dairy, cheese or butter. Technically, I was a pesco-vegetarian since I was eating dried codfish ("saltfish" in Jamaica) for a few weeks during the transition during which I substituted healthier alternatives to the destructive poisons I had been using all my life. (See substitution checklist in Resources.)

As a result of being a vegan and fit to breed advocate for now over 20 years, my energy level is higher; I thrive on less sleep; my sexual vitality is stronger; even my thoughts are clearer! In fact, I'm going to say that being vegan gave me the clarity and courage to quit my job, pursue my passion, and become a full-time "passionpreneur" and "nomadpreneur"—a decision that has taken me 8,000 miles to the other side of the world to find my bliss!

Now, I can't promise you the same results, I can only offer my experience as one example of how far being fit to breed has taken me. Your travel mileage may vary!

The Cures ▲

What works for me...and others!

37. ❏ Cure for the first time failure ❏

The simple cure for this is to accept that it happens, and not to get anxious about it beforehand if/when it does. A simple solution is to actually tell your partner about the first time failure phenomenon beforehand. That simple communication will do wonders to reduce the stress level and performance anxiety that can often accompany this situation.

38. ❏ Cure for incompatible DNA ❏

People enter into relationships for many reasons—from simple loneliness to financial security. Nature, however, is not concerned with bank account balances, or with what the neighbors think, or family bloodlines. Chemistry—that magnetic pull and electric attraction you feel—is Nature's way of fulfilling its directive. To start a relationship without this valid component of attraction is asking for trouble!

39. ❏ Cure for dating the wrong type ❏

The more clarity you achieve about what turns you on, the less likely you'll be to find yourself in a situation where you're not rising to the occasion. There should be no shame in pursuing the type you like. If you like short women with large feet, then accept it, embrace it, and seek them out!

40. ❏ Cure for the DOM/sub mismatch ❏

The more you embrace your DOM/sub wiring, and the more you seek out those with whom you are most compatible, the more satisfied you will be and less likely to find yourself struggling to keep the fire going. It is a misconception and unrealistic expectation to believe you can or should be able to be sexually compatible with everyone even if you are attracted to them and they to you!

41. ❏ Cure for being in the wrong society ❏

If the reason you're faltering is because your town, society or culture is not giving you what you want, then move! Yes, I know it's easier said that done, but I'll share a simple quote that is, in my opinion, the bottom line of this discussion:

"It takes far less effort to find and move to the society that has what you want than it does to try to reconstruct an existing society to match your standards." -Harry Browne, *How I Found Freedom in an Unfree World*

42. ❏ Cure for lack of fulfillment ❏

To find a greater level of fulfillment in life, start asking different questions. *Why am I here? What is the reason for my existence? What is my purpose? What is my passion? How can I use that passion in order to fulfill my purpose?* With those answers—or the quest for them—you can begin to fill the void that may be depriving your day-to-day life as well as your sex life of the necessary fulfillment. Take the passion personality test at www.passionprofit.com/itest

43. ❏ Cure for not being on the right team ❏

Fortunately, our society continues to change and grow and accept individuals who may have non-mainstream sexual orientations. The old maxim, "the truth shall set you free," is so appropriate. The more you (and our culture) embrace the truth of, and overcome the stigmas associated with your wiring, the freer you become to fully enjoy it!

44. ❑ Cure for tone deafness ❑

You can, with training and effort, move up the tone scale. The entire personal-growth/self-help industry is based on this possibility. You must embark on a mission of personal development in order to change the worldview and belief system that has you operating on lower levels of emotion. Don't be deaf to the fact that others, too, are operating at tones that may make *them* incompatible with *you*!

45. ❑ Cure for soul-specific sublimation ❑

This is not a "cure" but more a suggestion that you not feel there is something wrong with you if your actual desire for sex and intimacy has been curbed because your soul energy has been directed towards the accomplishment of some higher calling. Heed that calling, and you might find fulfillment and pleasure of an entirely different, even more satisfying type. It may even help reconcile previously competing aspects of your self-concept and magically improve your "impotence!"

46. ❑ Cure: Summary Chart ❑

Yes, if you know the cause of your impotence, then the cure is relatively simple, at least in theory. Here's a summary:

Cause	Cure
Classified as "unfit to breed" Bodily Toxicity and Depletion	Detox, cleanse and replenish using the Fit to Breed™ Protocol*
First time failure	Accept this is as common. May also be a result of incompatible DNA
Incompatible DNA	Don't force relationships in which there is no "chemistry"
Wrong "type"	Gain clarity about and pursue your "type"
Mismatched dom/sub	Man up
Wrong society	Get the heck outta Dodge!
Lack of fulfillment	Discover your passion
Not the right team	Embrace your orientation
Low on the Tone Scale	Move up the scale
Soul-specific sublimation	Embrace your soul age and pursue your purpose

*Before we proceed to the Fit to Breed™ Protocol, let's address a few myths and excuses people often use to distract themselves from their own success!

The Myths ▲

Debunking the conventional arguments

It's an odd quirk of human behavior that people often choose laziness, then seek to find justification for that laziness. In other words, rather than accept a challenging solution to their situation, they'd rather choose the easy way out, and then present platitudes (as excuses) in order to rationalize and justify it. Here are some of the most common excuses I hear when people are simply not up to the challenge of radically changing their behavior in order to achieve health:

47. ❏ Myth: "All things in moderation!" ❏

People who choose this excuse simply wish to keep practicing all the bad habits (excess food and drink, poor food choices, etc.) while convincing themselves that if they simply do it "in moderation" that all will be well.

How much poison is a moderate amount? Poison, taken to any degree is still poison. You cannot poison yourself and expect to be healthy and fit to breed.

48. ❏ Myth: "Everybody is different!" ❏

No. That is incorrect. Every human body is, in fact, essentially the same. All the cars come off the assembly line according to a specific design. The differences come with how we treat it once we own it. Ten years later, mine gets better gas mileage because of the fuel I chose. Mine *looks* better because I took better care of it. Your exhaust pipe is clogged, so mine performs better! However, the mechanics of how it operates— gas, oil, engine, pistons, transmission—everything is the same.

Similarly, when it comes to our bodies, the differences come about after time as a result of our deviation from the natural norm. The fact that your body rejects vegetables, for instance, is not because your body was somehow constructed differently from the 7 billion other bodies of the species. When your body rejects natural, organic food, it is not because you are so different from the other humans. It is not because there is something wrong with the food. No, there is something wrong with *you*, but it's not in your design. It's as a result of the distraction, delusions, diversions and departure from the natural norm that have defined your lifestyle.

It's because over time, perhaps over generations due to habits and the internal pollution inherited from your parents— your body is now functioning sub optimally. But that's not an indication that you are some sort of alien species for whom these principles do not apply. It means, simply, that you have some work to do in order to return the operation of your body to the way it was meant to perform.

Yes, we are all *designed* the same. Sperm meets with egg. Gestation, development and birth are all the same. Internal organs all function the same way. The slight variations in eye color, hair length and bone density are not major. If everyone were *really* different, Nature's principles couldn't work. The truth is, we are NOT all different. We are all the same.

49. ❑ Excuse: "I don't like vegetables!" ❑

Yes, I've met adults who use this as a reason they can't become vegetarian. To them I say: you've been led to believe you have a choice in the matter. You don't. That's like saying, "I don't really like air." The body was made to function on fruits and vegetables, not pizza, cola and hamburgers. It's that simple. Grow up.

50. ❑ Myth: "It's a matter of opinion" ❑

We can't move forward as a society if we keep asking questions we already know the answers to.
Fluoride? "What do you think? What's your opinion?"
Vaccines? "What do you think? What's your opinion?"
Climate change? "What do you think? What's your opinion?"
This tactic is often used in political debates. An issue is framed as a "debate" with opposing sides of supposedly equal merit. Well, the truth is, opinions may be divided, but reality is beyond debate. Some opinions are simply not valid. There comes a point when people must move beyond the fallacy of debate, and simply start acting from positions of truth.

For example, we're not there yet, but it will soon become commonly accepted that fluoride is a poison that should not be consumed, that certain vaccines cause autism, that cell phone use causes cancer, and that climate change is a reality. The fact that people cast themselves on either side of an imaginary debate does not lessen the severity of the damage that is being caused. It does not reduce the reality. Every time an issue is presented as a debate, and every time questions are asked in that "what's your opinion" way, it keeps us going backwards and stuck at zero.

The truth is, if you're practicing the Standard American Diet (SAD), practically everything you've been led to believe to be "food" is actually poisoning your body and making you unfit to breed. There IS no debate about this. You can be your own authority and decide on this now, or you can keep going back to zero every time a news report of a new study (sponsored by the Dairy Council) tells you that milk does a body good. The sooner you move beyond debate, the sooner you can reach a place where you're enjoying the benefits of being fit to breed.

It doesn't matter what anyone else's new study or opinion shows. Make your own decision, take a stance, establish your position once, right now, based on common sense, logic, critical analysis, even your own personal research using your own body, and then move forward.

If you wish to argue on behalf of your limitations and excesses, or if you wish to immerse yourself in a non-existent debate, then the ideas and suggestions in this manual will not work for you. You must be willing to move in the direction of change in order to achieve what you desire. Perhaps, what you need is simply the right motivation.

The Motivation▴

Here's what she said to me!

51. ❑ Motivation: "Where this power come from?" ❑

One night, my girl—whose native language is not English—grasped "it" after it had been doing its job for the previous hour, and with a look of puzzlement and ecstasy, started at it and asked, "Where this power come from?"

Now, perhaps it's just me, but I'm a pleaser, and so reviews like that help me to find the discipline to maintain my fit to breed lifestyle. Knowing I've got the vitality and "power" to satisfy my girl is a great motivator. (When they say women are attracted to power, this is what they mean!) There's also the ego-satisfaction of being called a "master!" There's the thrill of being able to live out my fantasies. There's the enjoyment of being able to have "porno quality" (multi-orgasmic, infinite duration) sex. Perhaps it's just a fear of "getting old."

In any case, in the same way I can't promise you the same results as I've had on the Fit to Breed Protocol, I cannot likewise predict what will serve as *your* motivation to embark upon and maintain it. You've got to find that on your own. Somewhere deep inside you, or perhaps from a source outside of you, you must find the motivation, to do what is necessary to be fit to breed forever!

52. ❑ Requirement: new thoughts ❑

Now then, even with the best motivations, it will still require a few things in order to succeed. Gandhi reportedly said, "You can't solve a problem with the same level of thinking that caused the problem in the first place," or words to that effect. Similarly, when it comes to your health, you are unfit to breed because of a certain way of thinking (and behaving). You cannot undo and reverse your condition using the same thoughts and behavior that created it. Something needs to change.

The fact that it may seem like a lot to have to remember, a lot to have to change, or a lot to sustain is nothing more than a testament to how far removed we as a society have become from natural, more health-supporting behaviors. The new thoughts and behaviors themselves are not difficult to implement, they are simply difficult to transition into if all you've known is their complete opposite.

To the same degree that you were once unconscious, inattentive to details, and immersed in immediate gratification; to that same degree must you now act consciously, pay attention to details and delay your gratification in order to achieve and sustain the condition of fit to breed. Nothing else will work.

We live in an aberrant paradigm, and part of creating health in an insanely aberrant paradigm such as ours requires getting over your fears as well as your addiction to comfort. Sometimes you must eat things that are not pleasant, and do things that are a little uncomfortable in order to reverse a lifetime of immediate gratification and lack of restraint. Your belief that there should be an *easy* way to do things is what has caused the condition in the first place. New thought is required.

53. ❏ Requirement: Courage and discipline ❏

Many people will try to sell you quick and easy strategies to do just about anything in life—everything from losing weight to making money, to having a better sex life. They will claim to have the magic pill or fairy dust that will work like a charm. Certain processes may, in fact, be simple. Specific techniques may be easy. Unique strategies may work like magic. Certain environments may be more conducive to success. However, there is often something missing from these formulas: how do you sustain the motivation?

It is my experience that you can achieve just about anything you desire in life if you have courage and discipline.

Once you are *introduced* to a new reality with a different set of choices, required actions, consequences and benefits, it requires *courage* to choose and embark on that reality in the face of *inertia and fear.*

Once you then *embark* on the new reality with its different set of choices, required actions, consequences and benefits, it requires *discipline* to maintain and sustain those actions in the face of *distraction and derision.*

Courage is discipline in the face of fear.

Discipline is courage in the face of distraction.

Courage and discipline are the interchangeable, complementary and inextricably linked sides of the same coin. Any solution that suggests otherwise is doing you a disservice.

With that said, becoming fit to breed requires:

The courage to (re)define yourself and your world view

The courage to embrace and act out your true wiring.

The courage to pursue the type of partner you are attracted to.

The courage to live outside the usual paradigm.
The discipline to choose real food for sustenance.
The discipline to fast for an extended period.
The discipline to delay gratification.

That's what all success boils down to: the courage and discipline to sustain your motivation. It cannot be given to you. It cannot be taught. It can only be suggested or inspired, but ultimately, *you* must find within yourself the courage to start, and the discipline to continue. That, in my opinion, and experience, is what is required to be fit to breed....forever!

54. ❑ Confession ❑

Having said that, I fully realize that this is not a mass-market book. This is not a book that huge segments of the public will be able to implement much less even appreciate. So, if you consider yourself just like everybody else, then do not attempt to use this book or implement the protocol. If you've already purchased this book, please request your money back. This book is for people who wish to stand out from the crowd. This book is for people who understand there will usually be a price to pay for anything of real and lasting value.

As I always say when it comes to real success: "If it were easy, everybody would be doing it!"

If it were easy to simply flip a switch and become fit to breed, everybody would be.

The "price" to pay, or at least the requirement for entry into this exclusive Fit to Breed club is courage and discipline.

If you believe you have that courage and discipline, then you're ready for the next step!

The Protocol ▲

A Daily Routine

Now that we've identified the major challenge, offered a new paradigm for understanding it, explored the causes, suggested some cures, debunked a few myths, found the motivation, and are prepared for what it will really require to succeed, now it's time to embark on a proven plan to achieve our objective! It's time to execute the Fit to Breed Protocol!

55. ❏ Super Prime Directive #1: Put it back! ❏

The significant difference between male and female orgasms is that men release and "lose" something during orgasm while women typically do not.* As a man, you lose semen along with nutrients and hormones each time you ejaculate. (Some say you also lose a little of your vital energy (chi) each time you ejaculate.) Now, you may only be able to *conserve* your chi, but you can and should "put back" the nutrients you lose (see "Chemical composition of semen" next page) Now, you don't have to be a Chemistry major to do this. Simply know that in order to be fit to breed, you must replace this loss and create an environment that is conducive to producing more viable sperm/semen.

For women there is depletion of kidney energy during sex, and a loss of iron each menstrual cycle. There is also female ejaculation (squirting).

56. ❏ Fact: Chemical composition of semen ❏

(_)= approximate amounts in mg per 100mL

ascorbic acid[1]	glucose (102mg)	pyruvic acid [9]
antigens	glutathione[4]	protein (5.04g)
biocarbonate[2]	hyaluronidase[5]	sodium[10] (300mg)
calcium (27.6mg)	inositol[6]	sorbitol[11]
chloride (142mg)	lactic acid (62g)	urea[12] (45g)
cholesterol	magnesium (11mg)	uric acid[13]
enzymes	nitrogen	vitamin B12
citric acid (528mg)	phosphate	water
creatine	phosphorus	zinc (16.5g)
DNA[3]	potassium (109mg)	
Fructose (272mg)	purine[7]	
	pyrimidin[8]	

(1) vitamin C
(2) biocarbonate buffers are bases
(3) deoxyribonucleic acid
(4) an important protein that kills free radicals
(5) protein that breaks-up acid, lowers the viscosity and increase the permeability of connective tissue and promotes the absorption of fluids
(6) an alcohol; a component of vitamin B
(7) special alkalies or bases (when mixed with acids create types of salt)
(8) an organic compound that causes the smell of semen
(9) a colorless acid that aids in metabolism or fermentation
(10) pure salt
(11) a sugar alcohol (sweetener) with 4 calories per gram
(12) the chief solid component of mammalian urine
(13) tasteless, odorless crystalline product of protein metabolism; also present in blood and urine

1% of ejaculate contains 100-600 million sperm The 99% protect, feed and fuel the sperm to their ultimate destination.

The protein content of the average amount of semen ejaculated is equivalent to that found in the white of a large egg.

Not surprisingly, calcium, phosphorus, sodium, potassium, magnesium and chlorine are also present in human breast milk.

Of the minerals lost, zinc is highest in concentration.

57. ❏ Directive: Maintain alkalinity ❏

Scientists use a measurement called the "pH scale" for measuring the acidity or alkalinity of various substances. (The letters pH mean power of Hydrogen). The pH scale ranges from 0 to 14. Lower numbers indicate a more acidic concentration and higher numbers are more alkaline, with 7 (the pH of pure water) being the neutral midpoint. The ideal pH of the human body is not 7, but is actually 7.365 (above neutral/slightly alkaline). Once outside of this range (either too acidic, or even too alkaline), the body's metabolism goes out of balance. Most people in our society—as a result of consuming sugar, meat, dairy, fried foods, etc.—are extremely acidic..

A prime directive on the Fit to Breed protocol, therefore, is to eat those foods, take those supplements and maintain a lifestyle that help to maintain an alkaline environment within the body. See the chart of acid vs. alkaline foods in Resources.

58. ❏ Directive: Keep the flow going ❏

Make sure there is consistent outflow of matter to match the inflow, and that nothing remains stuck inside the body that should be outside the body. The number of daily bowel movements should at least equal the number of times you eat per day. Now, it's best if your body does this naturally, but sometimes it may be necessary to help it along with enemas or colonics or salt water washes or bulking agents like fiber. Don't let the sun set on a blocked system. You'll notice an increase in sexual vitality and virility as you start having more bowel movements each day. Following is a technical explanation why.

59. ❑ Formula: A simple formula for Virility ❑

To get the most from any engine, it's not the amount or even the quality of fuel that matters most, it's the efficiency of the engine! Two engines can use the same amount and quality of fuel—say one gallon of gas—and one engine will travel 23 miles, while the other, more efficient engine will travel 50!

Similarly, your performance is based on your body's efficiency. So, how does one create an efficient, virile *human* sexual engine? Well, here's the formula adapted from Arnold Ehret's *Mucusless Diet & Healing System:*

The formula is: $V = P^2 - O$

"V" is for VIRILITY.

"P^2" is the POWER-POTENTIAL that drives the human machinery, keeps you alive, and gives strength and endurance.

"O" is OBSTRUCTION—foreign matter, mucus and anything that hinders circulation, the function of the organs, and flow. In another word, blockage. In words, the formula is:

Virility = Potential Power minus Obstruction

Hypothetically, let's say you have 100 imaginary units of potential power (P^2) in your body, but you also have 25 units of obstruction (O) in your colon. Therefore, the amount of virility your body has available to spend for sex is only 75.

$100(P^2)$otentialpower $- 25(O)$bstruction $= 75(V)$irility

You can see by this equation that as soon as "O" becomes *greater* than "P^2" the human machine must come to a standstill. Yes, $V = P^2 - O$ is the formula of life and virility, and at the same time you may call it the formula of impotence, illness and death.

60. ❑ Directive: Keep your body clean and pure❑

A clean engine is an efficient engine. A clean body is an efficient body. Every time you put something in or on your body that is not natural, you make it toxic to some degree. You should be conscious about reversing and compensating for those instances. For instance, if for some reason I eat a heavy meal late in the day (a no-no), or inadvertently eat something with wheat, sugar or some other ingredient I normally avoid, I will then fast for a 24-hour period the next day in order to allow the body time to reverse the effects of that overindulgence.

I also incorporate fasting, cleanses, detoxes, colonics, enemas and saunas in an effort to "reboot" and keep my body's operating system clean and pure. A clean cell never dies. (See *A Clean Cell Never Dies* for more!)

Fit to Breed Essentials

The strategy for achieving and sustaining these prime directives is to provide the body as much of a natural and pristine environment of sun, air, water, earth and food as possible. That's the secret! Remember: There's nothing man can devise that can be an improvement over nature in its original state.

61. ❑ Essential: Absorb sunshine ❑

The sun's ultraviolet rays are antiseptic and can kill bacteria, viruses, fungi, yeasts, molds, and mites in air and water, and on surfaces including our skin; convert cholesterol in the skin to Vitamin D; and regulate bodily processes. Infrared rays improve neuralgia, neuritis, arthritis, and sinusitis. Sunlight regulates hormones and bodily processes, stimulates the pineal gland, and normalizes heart rate, blood pressure and respiration;

increases oxygen to the blood and thus improves muscular endurance. Don't let "conventional wisdom" scare you away from soaking in the sun! Soak for at least one hour each day, shorter duration for people with paler, melanin-poor skin.

62. ❑ Essential: Drink water ❑

Simply drinking more and cleaner water can jump-start your body's cure of itself and immediately increase your energy. Purified, fluoride-free, chlorine-free room temperature rain water would be best. Fill a container with half-gallon to one gallon each day and drink throughout the day until complete.

63. ❑ Essential: Breathe oxygen ❑

It's been said that there was a time when the oxygen content in air was as high as 50%. Now it's less than 20% and worse in major cities. The more you can do to introduce oxygen into the system, the more optimally the body will function. Daily supplementation with food grade hydrogen peroxide ($H2O2$) actually increases oxygen uptake in the body. *(See H2O2 protocol in Resources.)*

64. ❑ Essential: Connect to the earth ❑

Think about this. In our modern world, and particularly in what Bob Marley called the "concrete jungle," it is possible for someone to be born, live and die without their feet ever touching the actual soil of the earth. From concrete tiles in the hospital, asphalt paved roads on the way home, shoes on the sidewalk, tiles and slippers and socks in the home or elevated high-rise apartment, sneakers in the playground, sandals on the beach, years can go by without ever experiencing the grounding and rejuvenating effect of actually connecting to the earth. I've found that simply running barefoot on the beach keeps the body grounded, and also increases the air intake, gets the blood pumping, and results in an increase in my libido.

Relearning Food

65. ❑ Relearning Food: What to eat ❑

Just because something can be chewed and swallowed does not make it real food. I define real food as *"unmodified, raw, enzyme-rich fruits and vegetables eaten in as close to their natural state as possible."* Canned carrots are not the same as fresh carrots. A boiled carrot is not the same as a fresh carrot. If you can't put it in the ground and grow another one, then it's not real food (generally speaking!) (See "The Carrot Conversation" on the Ageless Adept Blog: www.agelessadept.com/blog)

66. ❑ Relearning Food: When to eat ❑

Eating your heaviest meal during the daytime hours (12noon -3pm) when your energy level is highest will give your body time to digest and eliminate before going to bed.

67. ❑ Relearning Food: How often to eat ❑

Look around at the epidemic of obesity in our western societies. Common sense will tell you there's no way that eating *more* could be the answer to our society's health woes. Caloric restriction is the hallmark of the longest-lived and healthiest cultures around the world. Once your body has normalized, you'll find that "eat when hungry" means you'll actually eat less than you might be eating now.

68. ❑ Relearning Food: Why to eat ❑

The Fit to Breed concept of *why* to eat is probably a bit different from yours. I eat for more than just pleasure. That means I sometimes eat things that I don't like, but that I know have a nourishing or purging effect on my body.

I think of every meal as medicine. I know that may not sound appetizing, but all that means is every time I prepare a meal, I take the opportunity to do something good for my system. I keep the following supplements on hand: DMSO, MSM, nutritional yeast, ionic minerals, blackstrap molasses, bee pollen, aloe vera, lecithin, sea weeds like kelp, dulse and Irish moss and I'll use these to 'nutrify' salads, soups, juices and shakes. Speaking of which:

69. ❑ Relearning Food: How to cook ❑

As I was preparing this revised edition of *Fit to Breed*, I got an email from a young lady who had a chance to spend time with me for a week here on Saipan. She's now returned to her home country, and emailed me.

She wrote: *"What condiments do you put on your veggies to make them taste so yummy? You've told me salt & cayenne before, but I use those and mine don't come out like yours. So 'fess up!"*

I replied: "If you can't replicate the taste exactly, don't worry about it too much. Yes, it could be something tangible like the spices, and even the flavor imparted by the history and residual flavors deep in the pots, but I think about my grandmother's cooking back in Jamaica, and I realize there is also something intangible that goes into each person's preparation. I knew she was the one who prepared my soup and dumplings, that she loved me and gave me 13 dumplings when no little 7 year old should be eating that many at one meal!

It's likely that the taste you recall comes from knowing that your man prepared it for you, that he cares about you and is feeding you to fatten you up for his and your pleasure later!

[It was then that I had the revelation]

"Ahh, just had an epiphany! When I cook for you, the underlying intention is to nourish and rejuvenate. It's not for taste. (I know it will taste good because I know how to cook, but that's not my focus). My focus is on repair, reversal, rejuvenation and regeneration. As I put every item in the CockTale or in the prepared dishes, I'm aware of the therapeutic benefit of each one, and that benefit comes to the forefront of my mind, and I envision it having that effect in you."

She replied: "*Wow! I think you have just clarified it all. I have always maintained that cooking for someone is truly an act of love and that each cook brings their own "sabor" to it that is unique because of who they are—but it never occurred to me that the chef's "intent" could be one of the most important ingredients. Your food really did rejuvenate, repair, reverse and regenerate me...*Not only did it taste good, I could feel how good it was for me!"

The bottom line: cook with "fit to breed" intention!

Best Practices

70. ❏ Practice: Sleep ❏

You may find you want to sleep more during the initial phases of the protocol. During sleep is when the body rests, reverses and rejuvenates. You must carve time in your schedule for sufficient hours of sleep especially in the beginning.

71. ❏ Practice: Exercise ❏

Weak muscle energy is one cause of impotence. Physical activity is one sure way to increase libido. Rebounding is a very therapeutic activity.

72. ❏ Practice: The 5 Rites ❏

As described in Ancient Secrets of the Fountain of Youth, there are "five ancient Tibetan rites which hold the key to lasting youth, health, and vitality. For thousands of years these seemingly magical rites were shrouded in secrecy in remote Himalayan monasteries."

The title of the original publication is The Eye of Revelation by Peter Kelder and may be in the public domain. A free version of just the 5 rites (plus warm up exercises) can be found at http://www.mkprojects.com/pf_TibetanRites.htm

73. ❏ Practice: Cleaning the blood ❏

Many ailments, including many skin conditions (i.e. carbuncles, blackheads, pimples), are simply the result of impure blood. Woodroot tonic, Echinacea, Burdock, Dandelion, Sarsaparilla and certain tissue salts aid in cleansing toxins from the bloodstream. Make a regular practice of drinking teas and taking these supplements in order to cleanse the blood. Strong blood is a requirement for virility and is one of the causes of impotence.

74. ❑ Practice: Deer exercise ❑

The Deer Exercise for men, as described by Dr. Stephen T. Chang in The Tao of Sexology, is a two-part exercise designed for sexual and spiritual rejuvenation. It was developed thousands of years ago by Taoist sages who observed actual deer in the wild. It builds the tissues of the sex organs, increases sexual energy, and protects the prostate.

The first part of the exercise involves cupping the testicles in the palm of one warmed hand, and then rubbing the pubic area just below the navel in a circular motion with the other hand 81 times. Switch hands and rub in the opposite direction. In the second part of the Deer Exercise, you repeatedly "tighten the muscles around your anus and draw them up and in" and hold as long as you can. Stop and relax, and repeat as often as you can.

Tip: When you urinate, attempt to stop and release the stream of urine. You'll be using the same muscles and will be able to determine how the Deer Exercise is working.

According to Chang, the exercise strengthens the prostate and can correct premature ejaculation, low hormone levels, testicular infections, wet dreams and impotence---most of which are related to poor prostate function.

The exercise can be done throughout the day at any time (standing, sitting or lying down) as well as *immediately* prior to intercourse (for premature ejaculation), and even *during* intercourse to improve endurance. Remember to "go in relaxed, pull out tight" (penetrate the vagina with your muscles relaxed, but tighten your muscles as you pull out.)

75. ❑ Practice: Prostate Massage ❑

In addition to a manual finger massage (insert finger in rectum and massage prostate; see diagram for location), the Deer Exercise also massages the prostate internally.

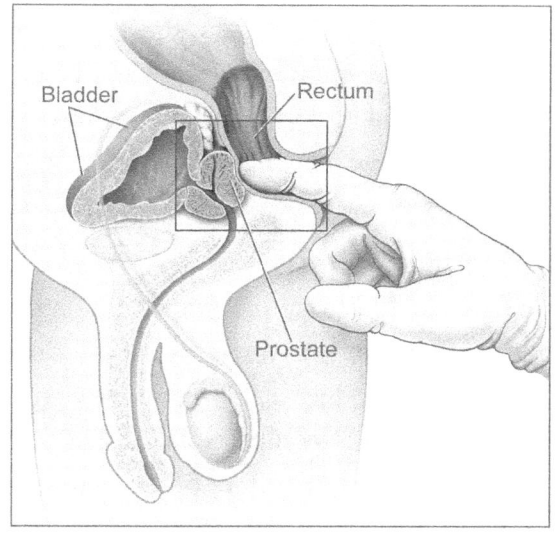

Image released by the National Cancer Institute

For more detailed instructions, read *The Tao of Sexology*

Detoxes, Cleanses & Fasts
⌀ = those I have NOT personally tried.

76. ❑ Detox: colonics ❑

While lying on your back on a special table, water is introduced into the rectum and repeatedly floods then evacuates the colon. My first colonic experience was 7 days of a daily colonic, supplemented with green juice and clay and psyllium throughout the day. At the time, I had already been vegan for about 10 years and felt I only needed a single day's colonic evacuation. I reluctantly agreed to the 7-day program at the insistence of my hygienist. On the fourth day, the worms came out! I'll spare you the photos! Guess she knew what she was doing, after all! Sure, there are other ways to get at those pesky worms that may be lodged deep in your colon, but I swear by colonics because of my own positive experience!

77. ❑ Detox: Coffee enemas ❑

Coffee enemas detoxify the liver, stimulating both liver and gallbladder to remove toxins, open bile ducts, increase peristaltic action, and produce enzyme activity for healthy red blood cell formation and oxygen uptake. The coffee enema flushes the liver of toxins. The effect of your first coffee enema is immediate, unmistakable, rejuvenating and life changing
Instructions: http://agelessadept.com/resources/coffee

78. ❑ Detox: Skin Scrub ❑

Pounds of toxins can be removed by brushing the skin with a loofah brush.

79. ❑ Detox: Multi-Day detoxes ❑

There are several brands of 7-day, 10-day, 14/28-day cleanses designed to clean the colon as well as other bodily systems. I've tried Arise and Shine™ and TheCleaner.com. Be sure to follow the directions closely, and drink plenty of water especially if you're using a cleanse that includes clay.

80. ❑ Cleanse: Organ-specific cleanses ❑

Dr. Hulda Clark's liver cleanse, parasite cleanse, kidney cleanse and more are available at http://www.drclark.net/ as well as through her family's official site at http://www.drclarkstore.com/

81. ❑ Cleanse: Zapper protocols ❑

Zappers send an electrical charge through the blood that kills hard to reach parasites. Continued use gets at their larvae so the body is not repopulated. I've used Sota Instruments™ brand as well as the Ultimate Zapper™ from Canada.

82. ❑ Detox: Dry sauna ❑

A dry sauna increases circulation and stimulates sweating forcing toxins out of the body. I find I need at least a few hours of recuperation time after a sauna, so I do it a day or two before a play date. The type of sauna I do is a detox sauna that can purge the body of heavy metals and other toxins.
Instructions: http://agelessadept.com/resources/sauna.pdf

83. ❑ Fast: Fast and grow young ❑

Fasting is Nature's first cure, and is perhaps the best way to allow the body the time it needs to truly heal. Many people report increasing, not decreasing energy, mental clarity, and a

reversal of chronic conditions the longer they fasts
See Fast & Grow Young at www.fastandgrowyoung.com

84. ❑ Fast: Master Cleanse ❑

Also called the "lemonade diet," this is a great fast for beginners. It requires lemons, water, maple syrup and cayenne pepper. Purchase *The Master Cleanser* by Stanley Burroughs and follow the instructions. Many support websites exist online.

85. ❑ Cleanse: Oil pulling ❑

Oil pulling is the practice of taking about an ounce of oil--typically sesame or coconut oil--swishing it around the mouth and "pulling" it through and around the teeth for about 10-20 minutes. Dating back to around 500 BC, the practice is called Kavala or Gandusha, and is said to cure some 30 systemic diseases such as headache, migraine, eczema, diabetes and asthma. The premise is that the oil "pulls" toxins out of the body. It has been used extensively for whitening teeth, and preventing tooth decay, treating bad breath, bleeding gums, dryness of throat, cracked lips and for strengthening teeth, gums and the jaw. Research online for more details.

Supplements: The Usual Suspects

Search and you'll find erection enhancers, libido lifters, herbal helpers, and augmenting aphrodisiacs containing some or all of the following. Entire books can be and have been written about each. Research any side effects before using.

⌀ = products/herbs I've NOT personally tried.

86. ❑ Supplement: ⌀ Bioperine ❑

Research shows when Chrysin is combined with Piperine (aka Bioperine), men see reductions in blood estrogen levels and increases in free testosterone in as little as 30 days. (20mg)

87. ❑ Supplement: ⌀ Choline ❑

Acetylcholine or ACh is the neurotransmitter that sends signals from the brain to the penis. Increase ACh (by taking Choline), and sex drive goes up. Users recommend Choline plus vitamin B5 (or B-5 alone for endurance) about 20-30 minutes before sex for the full effect from the start. (1000mg)

88. ❑ Supplement: ⌀ Chrysin ❑

A flavenoid found in honey, propolis and plants. Bodybuilders take chrysin supplements to increase available testosterone, in part through reducing the conversion of testosterone into estrogen. Also an antioxidant and reduces anxiety and stress. (1500mg)

89. ❑ Herb: Damiana ❑

A liquor made from Damiana leaves has been used as an aphrodisiac and to boost sexual potency by natives of Mexico, including the Mayans, and for male *and* female sexual stimulation. It is used to increase energy, treat asthma, menstrual problems, constipation, anxiety, mild depression, impotence and brings oxygen to the genital area. In studies, extracts of Damiana sped up the mating behavior of "sexually sluggish" (impotent) male rats, but had no effect on normal rats.

90. ❑ Herb: Ginseng ❑

An "adaptagen" (adapts to the body's needs and goes where it's needed); promotes energy, appetite, female fertility; regulates hormonal functions, cholesterol, fat levels and nervous system; enhances mental function, nerve growth, resistance, endurance, life expectancy, menses; eases childbirth and treats periodontal disease.

91. ❑ Herb: Horny Goat Weed ❑

Used in traditional Chinese medicine (TCM) to treat various sexual dysfunctions, osteoporosis, hypertension, bronchitis, heart disease, polio and more.

92. ❑ Herb: ⌧ Kava Kava ❑

Painkiller used by indigenous Pacific islanders (Polynesia, Micronesia, Hawaii) for arthritis; reduces chronic pain, menstrual discomfort, tension in muscles, asthma and urinary tract infections. Relieves stress due to social anxiety.

93. ❑ Supplement: L-arginine ❑

A non-essential amino acid found in food. Increases blood flow to the genitals. (2000-4000mg)

94. ❑ Herb: ℘ Nettle root ❑

In some men, "free" testosterone often binds with a protein known as "sex hormone binding globulin" (SHBG) and, as a result, testosterone is not available for sexual function. Nettle root binds with SHBG so the testosterone is freed.

95. ❑ Herb: ℘ Muira Puama ❑

Long used in England; increases blood flow to pelvic area, aiding erections in men and sensation and orgasm in women. Longterm use enhances production of sex hormones in both sexes. (750mg)

96. ❑ Herb: ℘ Norway Spruce ❑

Increasing estrogen levels in aging men are believed to contribute to prostate enlargement and prostate cancer. Enterolactone, a substance created in the body when Norway Spruce is processed, kills cancer cells in the prostate and reduces estrogen levels. (30mg)

97. ❑ Herb: ℘ Rhodiola ❑

Adaptagen; treats Parkinson's and Alzheimers, rejuvenates; boosts endurance; enhances memory, concentration; protects heart, liver; improves iron absorption; prevents prostate cancer; reduces stress, depression; increases appetite; improves sexual function and libido (with maca), restores desire to exercise

98. ❑ Herb: ℘ Tribulus ❑

Long history of use in traditional Chinese medicine and

Indian Ayurvedic practice; enhances sexual desire in men *and* women; increases testosterone, sex drive; erectile dysfunction.

99. ❑ Herb: Yohimbe ❑

Derived from the bark of the West African evergreen tree; used for centuries by men *and* women in traditional African medicine. Increases libido and stamina; improves erectile dysfunction, sexual sensation and orgasms. Dilates blood vessels, lowers blood pressure and carries blood to the genitals.

My Personal Arsenal
The daily routine. Use this as your shopping list!

100. ❑ Herb: Ashwagandha ❑

Used in Indian Ayurvedic medicine for over 3,000 years; promotes sleep; regulates the thyroid; enhances immunity; balances the nervous system; combats diabetes; restores vitality; reduces constipation; builds the liver, and is an aphrodisiac that stimulates the libido, renews sperm, eases menopause symptoms and painful periods, reverses infertility, premature ejaculation, cures impotence, and restores the strength of the horse (*ashwagandha* means "smell of the horse").

101. ❑ Supplement: Black seed oil ❑

Ancient panacea for ulcers, diarrhea, asthma, flu and more. Use topically for pain and skin conditions. Use in juices, smoothies and shakes. Good for male impotence.

102. ❏ Supplement: Vitamin C ❏

With so many benefits, it should have been called Vitamin #1 rather than the third letter in the alphabet! An antioxidant that strengthens the heart, builds immunity, clears bacteria, reduces cellular DNA damage, helps iron absorption, strengthens hair, delays signs of aging and more!

103. ❏ Supplement: Chlorophyll ❏

Deodorizes the body. Removes effects of pollution. Increases peristaltic action and relieves constipation. Regenerates damaged liver cells, increases circulation to all organs by dilating blood vessels; Include in green juices.

104. ❏ Supplement: Colloidal Silver ❏

Alkaline. Natural antibiotic; Kills 650 organisms; Helps destroy bacteria, fungi and viruses (antibiotics are effective only against about 12 forms of bacteria and fungi, not viruses); Helpful against acne, allergies, arthritis, athlete's foot, boils, burns, candida, cystitis, diabetes, eczema, hay fever, parasitic infections, psoriasis, ringworm, warts, and yeast infections.

105. ❏ Supplement: DMSO ❏

DMSO, or dimethyl sulphoxide, is a by-product of papermaking. It is colorless industrial solvent and was first identified in 1866 by a Russian scientist. It heals scars, keloids and burns, improves eyesight, eases pain, helps with stroke, heart attacks, arthritis; reduces pain, helps with cancer, diabetes, sinusitis, herpes and more. Use topically and include it in green juices. Check out the book, *DMSO* by Morton Walker and view this article about its many amazing benefits:

www.sott.net/article/228453-DMSO-The-Real-Miracle-Solution

106. ❑ Supplement: Grapefruit seed extract ❑

Broad spectrum treatment for viruses, bacteria, fungi and parasites. One of the best alkalizers. Stimulates immune system. Useful for skin conditions, gum disease, diarrhea, chronic fatigue, water purification, salmonella. You'll find that anything that alkalizes the body has an almost immediate energy-boosting effect. Put a few drops in juices and smoothies.

107. ❑ Supplement: Green powder mix ❑

Blend of various greens, vitamins, minerals, antioxidants, fiber, fruits, enzymes and probiotics in powder form. Green Vibrance™ is very popular. I currently use Greens Pak by Trace Minerals®. Use in Power CockTale (see Recipes)

108. ❑Supplement: Hydrogen peroxide (Food grade) ❑

Ingesting H202 orally delivers oxygen to the body. Similar therapies (ozone, ozonated water) give an immediate boost in energy. [See H202 Protocol in Resources]

109. ❑ Herb Tonic: Koromante bitters ❑

From the Koromante people of Africa. Traditionally used by the people of Africa, Caribbean and Latin America to clean the stomach, intestines and colon of waste matter and help relieve constipation. Drink alone for maximum benefit.

110. ❑ Herb Tonic: African "Manback" ❑

A combination of roots and barks from Ghana. Traditionally used for spine, nerves, male reproductive system weaknesses and impotence.

111. ❑ Supplement: MSM ❑

MSM (methyl-sulphony-methane, or dimethyl sulphone) is organic sulphur. Along with related compounds, DMSO and DMS, are the sources of nearly all sulphur in the body, plants and animals. Sulphur ensures the proper functioning of various body processes, healthy skin, nails and hair, and helps with cell repair and tissue/organ renewal. The highest amount of MSM is in breast milk. MSM in the body decreases over time. Use 2-10g/day to replenish and for therapeutic benefits.

112. ❑ Supplement: Niacin ❑

A critical ingredient for the detox sauna, Niacin accelerates the breaking down of fat to release toxins. Do not buy niacinamide or flush-free niacin. You want the flush!

113. ❑ Herb: Oil of oregano ❑

Antiviral, antibacterial, antifungal agent rivaling pharmaceutical antibiotics. Destroys organisms that contribute to skin infections and digestive problems. Strengthens immune system. Increases joint and muscle flexibility. Improves respiratory health. Stops infections (cold and flu). Fights yeast and fungi, allergies, hay fever and sinusitis.

114. ❑ Supplement: Probiotics ❑

Maintains the intestinal flora in the digestive tract to digest, utilize and eliminate food.

115. ❑ Supplement: Tissue salts ❑
Mineral salts essential for the body's optimal function.

116. ❑ Supplement: Trace minerals ❑
Restores the depletion of up to 72 essential and trace minerals necessary for the body's optimal functioning.

117. ❑ Herb Tonic: Jamaican Woodroot ❑
Passed down by the fierce Maroons. Used traditionally in Jamaica for generations. Includes herbs (eg. Strong Back, Four Man's Strength), that cleanse the blood, eliminate toxins, mucous and waste; corrects and normalizes digestive and gastrointestinal disorders, circulation, heart and blood pressure, body weight, brain and nervous system, liver, lymphatic and glandular systems, kidney and bladder function and impotence.

118. ❑ Supplement: ☒Shilajit ❑
As of the writing of this 2020 edition, I'm about to order and try shilajit. hilajit or mumijo is a blackish-brown powder or an exudate from high mountain rocks, often found in the Himalayas, Russia, and in the north of Chile, where it is called Andean Shilajit. It is a natural substance formed for centuries by the gradual decomposition of plants by the action of microorganisms. It contains fulvic acid and more than 84 minerals , so it offers numerous health benefits. It can function as an antioxidant to improve your body's immunity and

memory, an anti-inflammatory, an energy booster, and a diuretic to remove excess fluid from your body

Super Food list
Keep these on hand and incorporate them into cooking.

119. ❑ Food: Apple cider vinegar ❑
Promotes stamina; regulates cholesterol, metabolism; enhances immune system, digestion; cures skin conditions, acne, constipation, arthritis and gout; fights allergies, urinary tract infections, food poisoning; use in salads, Power CockTale.

120. ❑ Food: Barley grass powder ❑
Extremely alkaline; concentrated source of minerals, amino acids and vitamins including B12; inhibits cancer including prostate, leukemia, brain tumors; promotes digestion, age reversal, heart health, weight loss; eases arthritis, ulcers; source of chlorophyll. Include in green juices.

121. ❑ Food: Bee pollen (and raw honey) ❑
One of nature's most complete foods. Richest known source of vitamins, minerals, amino acids, hormones, enzymes and fats, natural antibiotics. Promotes growth of healthy new cells, tissue repair, toxin elimination, resistance to infections, fertility in women, calmness. Regulates cholesterol levels, blood pressure, nervous system. Enhances sexual activity,

memory, stamina, endurance. Combats cancer, diabetes, arthritis, depression. Use in cereal, yogurt and smoothies.

122. ❑ Food: Chlorella powder ❑

Used in Japan; highest amount of chlorophyll of any plant. balances cholesterol; Promotes good bacteria, energy; enhances digestion; eases constipation, ulcers, colitis; Fights infection, radiation; Treats fibromyalgia, cancer, radiation exposure; 60% protein, 18 amino acids, B12; use in green juices.

123. ❑ Food: Coconut oil (virgin) ❑

Promotes strong bones, weight loss, healthy hair; regulates digestion; enhances immunity, energy, mineral absorption; fights bacteria, fungi, viruses; very stable at high temperatures so is best oil for cooking; use for oil pulling, skin rejuvenation, sunblock, and daily supplement.

124. ❑ Food: Flax seed/oil ❑

First cultivated in Europe; source of Omega oils (3&6); promotes fertility, heart health; eases constipation, inflammation, gallstones, nerve damage; contains lignans which regulate hormones; helps prostate, infertility and impotence; Not for cooking. Use on rice and salads, take orally daily. The ground seeds make a good flour and fiber for constipation.

125. ❑ Food: Garlic ❑

Natural antibiotic and immune enhancer. Garlic's *allicin*

increases blood flow to genitals. Add raw to salads, last in stir fries and soups.

126. ❏ Food: Goji berries ❏

Also known as "Wolfberry," this fruit has been used in Asia for over 6000 years; promotes longevity; enhances immune function; fights cancer; increases fertility and male sexual function by improving circulation. Sprinkle on cereals. Use as tea. Add to smoothies.

127. ❏ Food: Irish moss (sea weed) ❏

Aka "carrageen moss" (Scien. names: *Chondrus crispus* or *Gracilaria*). Mineral-rich Gracilaria is boiled with cinnamon and milk to make a thick drink for male virility both in Trinidad & Tobago, as well as in Jamaica—where the drink is called "Put it Back!" Use in smoothies, soups and porridge.

128. ❏ Food: Kelp ❏

Provides iodine for efficient thyroid and pituitary function, iron, calcium, potassium, magnesium; Promotes weight loss, nail/hair growth; enhances immune system; fights off infection. Include in soups, salads. Add last to dishes.

129. ❏ Food: Lecithin ❏

Promotes cell permeability; regulates good/bad cholesterol; balances circulatory and nervous systems; reverses heart disease; enhances brain/memory function; fights atherosclerosis; repairs liver damage due to alcohol. Available as soy lecithin. Sprinkle on salads.

130. ❏ Food: Nutritional yeast: ❏

Provides B vitamins (sometimes B12), trace minerals, protein, all 18 amino acids; enhances energy, memory; free of dairy, soy, gluten and sugar and animal products; will not aggravate a Candida condition. Some people like its cheesy flavor on popcorn. Sprinkle on salads, rice, quinoa.

131. ❏ Food: Maca powder ❏

Cultivated in Peru as an aphrodisiac for over 3000 years; increases energy; improves fertility; regulates hormones; reduces depression; enhances mental clarity; reduces anxiety; improves circulation; builds muscle, improves skin tone, promotes hair growth, thyroid function; increases libido/sexual function for men and women Use in smoothies and shakes, sprinkle on fruit. Use in CockTale (see Recipes) (300mg)

132. ❑ Food: Malunggay ❑

Aka Moringa Oleifera; provides 90+ vitamins, minerals and phytonutrients, over 46 antioxidants, 36 anti-inflammatory compounds. 7 times the vitamin C of oranges, 4 times the vitamin A of carrots, 4 times the calcium of milk, 3 times the potassium of bananas and 2 times the protein of yogurt; contains 18 amino acids, including eight essential.

133. ❑ Food: Olive oil ❑

Provides unsaturated fat, omega-3 fatty acids; balances cholesterol levels; reduces inflammation; prevents heart disease, prostate tumors, lowers blood sugar; skin moisturizer. Use for salads and to pour on rice or grains. Do not use for cooking.

134. ❑ Food: Pumpkin seeds ❑

Discovered in Mexican caves dating 7,000 BC, and used in ancient Greece; provide copper, iron, manganese, magnesium and phosphorus and protein; lower cholesterol levels; prevent osteoporosis and kidney stones; fight prostate cancer; combat tapeworms and parasites and arthritis; One of the best natural sources of zinc. Use in smoothies, grind and add to coleslaw.

135. ❑ Food: Royal Jelly ❑

Traditional Chinese medicine; provides vitamins, minerals, proteins antioxidants; boosts strength, energy; promotes hormonal balance in men and women; enhances concentration, brain function; fights insomnia; repairs bones, nails, hair; combats impotence, frigidity; improves endurance, resistance to viruses bacteria; restores apetite; stimulates libido.

136. ❑ Food: Spirulina powder ❑

Perhaps the most nutritionally complete of all food supplements, provides protein, complex carbohydrates, iron, vitamins A, K, and B complex, beta carotene and antioxidants; rich in chlorophyll, lipids, fatty nucleic acids, iron, magnesium and trace minerals, B12, gamma-linolenic acid (a compound in breast milk); promotes digestion and bowel function; enhances eyesight; builds muscle; increases stamina; stimulates intestinal flora; combats cellular degeneration, radiation sickness; improves absorption; reduces bad cholesterol. Provides 8 essential/10 non-essential amino acids (incl. Arginine: seminal fluid is 80% Arginine.) plus zinc; Detoxifies the blood. Use in salads, juices, smoothies, shakes; sprinkle on rice and grains.

137. ❑ Food: Watermelon rind ❑

Useful for healing mild erectile dysfunction as it contains citrulline, a blood vessel relaxer. Serves as a natural cure for increasing libido. Eat the white rind, and, after scraping off the outer layer of skin, use the rind for juicing.

Spices

138. ❑ Herb/Spice: Cayenne ❑

Warms the body. Good for the kidneys, lungs, spleen, pancreas, heart, and stomach; provides carotene, vitamins A, B1, B2, B3, B5, B6, B9, and C; promotes weight loss; enhances Immune system; fights Psoriasis; combats herpes, shingles, ulcers; A catalyst for all herbs, stimulates the appetite, aids digestion by stimulating gastric juices; reduces inflammation; increases blood flow to areas afflicted with rheumatism, arthritis; improves metabolism; relieves gas, colds, and stops bleeding from ulcers. Sprinkle on everything you can handle!

139. ❑ Herb/Spice: Cinnamon ❑

Helps with constipation, coronary problems, diarrhea, digestive irritation indigestion, nausea, parasites. Sprinkle on fruits and in porridges and smoothies.

140. ❑ Herb/Spice: Ginger ❑

Boosts circulation; cures indigestion; combats inflammation; improves arthritis, fevers, headaches, toothaches; prevents motion sickness, menstrual cramps; reduces bloating, heartburn, flatulence; suppresses cancer cells; Sprinkle on fruits and in porridge. Every meal should include some diced ginger.

141. ❑ Herb/Spice: Sea salt ❑

Find a brand with no additives and no added iodine. Use for your internal saltwater wash. (see Master Cleanser)

142. ❑ Food & Spices: Miscellaneous ❑
❑ Bananas provide bromelain and B vitamins
❑ Celery promotes *androsterone* an aphrodisiac in male sweat
❑ Avocados' folic acid and B6, a hormone regulator
❑ Asparagus is high in Vitamin E
❑ Chili peppers' *capsaicin* releases endorphis
❑ Basil increases sex drive and promotes fertility
❑ Figs are high in amino acids

The Play Date ▲
Where the rubber meets the road!

"Play Date" Logistics
A few tips for maximizing the intimacy and intensity!

143. ❑ Play Date: Eat less before sex ❑
On those days you know you'll be having sex, I'd advise eating a light meal early in the day or not at all. You'll be, in effect, taking the energy and blood flow the body would use for digestion, and diverting it to maintaining your erection. If you recall, part of the formula for efficient operation comes from reducing the encumbrances, not loading up on fuel.

You'd be better off taking green juices, shakes and the "comeback cocktale" rather than a heavy meal. Feast on your partner instead! Feed your hunger after the date!

144. ❑ Play Date: Enema before, eat after ❑

Performing a coffee enema, or a chlorophyll & H202 enema a few hours before your play date will have a tremendous effect on your vitality. Be sure you allow enough time for total evacuation to occur. Be careful you don't overdo this and end up depleting your lower colon of necessary minerals, or becoming dependent on enemas for regular bowel movements.

145. ❑ Play Date: The greatest secret of all! ❑

Now, this might be the greatest secret for remaining fit to breed forever. It may seem counterintuitive, especially if you view sex as a means to instant pleasure. The following is "Man Must" #2 (of the 7 things a man must provide his lover), excerpted from *"If you want to be my girlfriend..."* :

MAN MUST delay orgasm and last more than one hour

I once read an erotic story about a woman who took a new lover. The storyteller proceeded to chronicle the amazing sex they had, focusing on the many, many times the man ejaculated and filled the woman with his essence. As I read the story, I heard myself thinking: *No, no, no, that's wrong!! You've got to save it, man! Save it!*

Because of my own health beliefs, I came to the conclusion many years ago that I didn't want to expend my semen countless times over a lifetime of wanton, libidinous encounters. Having done that for many youthful years, I knew I always felt depleted afterwards —not just physically, but on a spiritual level as well. I recall learning from the *Tao of Sexology*, that much more than just a 'lovin' spoonful' of semen is lost during a man's ejaculation. In addition to the vitamins and minerals, there is a life force that is irretrievably spent. A friend once told me that you lose a piece of your spiritual being to each person you take to bed. Fanatic that I am about retaining my youthful essence, and spiritual purity, I now refrain from ejaculating when I have sex. As a result, I've noticed a marked improvement in my energy level, virility and desire for sex. I can go for hours at a time without climaxing, and thus maintain a higher level of arousal on days I'm not having sex. The sexual energy is retained, and remains available for me to sublimate it towards creative and business pursuits since that energy is not spent.

The drawback of this practice is that my girlfriends are deprived of the thrill of seeing me climax, as well as whatever benefit is derived from sharing the seed of my loins! What they all seem to agree upon, however, is that 2-4 hour marathon sex with someone who is fit to breed, who cares about their pleasure, and who offers a certain other "man must" (see #7) is a trade-off they're willing to make. For the record, I do let them experience my climax at least once a month. Their ego needs must be met and satisfied, too! [end excerpt]

Note: when I *do* decide to climax, I do not feel depleted and drained as I did in the past.

146. ❑ Play Date: Don't call it a comeback! ❑

You may think of the term, cycles, as relating to female menstruation, but men have cycles, too. The male cycle concerns the frequency of ejaculation.

I've mentioned throughout this manual the need to conserve one's semen depletion in order to optimize one's vital energy. I also mentioned the Truth of Rhythm that governs all things. According to Taoist principles, a man can "safely" ejaculate (meaning without over-depleting their vital energy) if they ejaculate in between their optimum ejaculation cycles— what I call your "comeback" time! To determine your cycle, ejaculate as normal, then commit to refraining from another ejaculation for as long as you can. When you reach the point where you feel you absolutely must have another ejaculation, note the number of days that have passed. This is your ejaculation cycle.

Keeping an "Ejaculation Log" (date, time) allows you to monitor the frequency of your ejaculations.

I highly recommend *The Tao of Sexology* for a more thorough and in-depth exploration of these principles, *plus* sexual positions that heal, techniques for increasing pleasure and more! *Fit to Breed* is a road map—what I like to think of as the "Breeder's Digest"—with "directions" to concepts that will require further study. This is definitely one of those concepts!

What if I actually WANT to breed?

Ooops! We've been focusing primarily on vitality, stamina and enjoyment of the sex itself, logistically. However, the title of this book is *Fit to Breed*, after all. So, here are some tips for men and women who actually *want* to breed!

147. ❑ Breed: What causes low sperm count? ❑

Here are some causes of low sperm count, lack of sperm motility (ability to move), and poor sperm morphology (shape):

☐ Electromagnetic frequencies (EMF) from cell phones and laptops
☐ Cigarette smoke
☐ Pesticides and hormones added to produce, dairy and meat
☐ Soy from genetically modified sources
☐ Alcohol consumption
☐ Plastics, when heated release estrogen-like substances
☐ Tight, restrictive clothing/underwear
☐ Stress

148. ❑ Breed: Increasing your "gonad nomads" ❑

Many of the nutrients and herbs experts recommend to increase production and motility for your little "semen seamen," "emission emissaries" or what I'm now calling "gonad nomads!" are already part of the Fit to Breed™ protocol: Zinc (in the seaweed and pumpkin seeds), Selenium (in the green powders, trace minerals and multivitamins), CoQ10, Vitamin E (Spirulina), Folic Acid (bee pollen), B12 (nutritional yeast), Vitamin C, L-Carnitine and antioxidants.

149. ❏ Breed: more tips for conceiving ❏

☐ Black Maca has been shown to increase sperm count and volume in men and Red Maca has been known to balance female hormones and ovulation cycles.

☐ Changes you make to your diet/lifestyle today will affect the sperm you ejaculate two to three months in the future

☐ Time your sex to roughly 12 -14 days after the first day of her period when she is ovulating and most fertile.

☐ Use sperm-friendly lubrication

☐ If trying to conceive, don't have sex standing up. It's harder for the sperm to reach the egg.

☐ Note: "female" sperm are heartier than male sperm, so having sex 2-4 days prior to ovulation will reportedly increase chances of having a girl since by the time ovulation occurs, the "male" sperm will already be dead. Similarly, having sex closer to the time of ovulation increases the chances of having a boy.

The Action ▲

The healing has begun

Now that we've outlined the prime directives, listed the essentials, relearned what/how/when/why to eat and cook, encouraged best practices, provided a list of supplements, herbs, tonics, and foods you'll need, and tips on how to optimize your evolving fit to breed status, now it's time to put everything in into action! Let the healing games begin! First, a few tips on what to expect, then we'll launch into action!

Quick Start: Overview

Here is a quick overview of how I would proceed, say, if I were coaching you through this. It includes what I would tell you to expect, as well as initial steps. When we get to the phase, remember, these are not separate, exclusive phases. All the suggested activities in each phase are typically happening at the same time. What changes is the focus.

150. ❏ Expect: Healing Crisis ❏

Once you start aligning yourself with truth, encouraging flow and eating real healing foods, your body will start to react —there will be elimination, detoxification, rebalancing, regeneration and rejuvenation as you start to reactivate your body's healing code and become fitter to breed.

As we learned, opposite conditions are just extreme ends of the same thing. Therefore, when your body starts to heal, you return back from illness along the same path that got you there, and you may actually re-experience some of the same pain and discomfort you experienced on the original journey.

In the case of detoxification, for instance, many of the toxins that are now lodged in your tissues will be loosened and find their way back into your bloodstream on their way to your kidneys and ultimately out of your system. That will result in certain symptoms of "illness" (headaches, pains) returning as you heal. In other words, you may feel worse while you're getting better. This is what we call a healing crisis.

151. ❏ Expect: Nature's pace ❏

Once you start the Fit to Breed Protocol, things will be happening inside your body of which you may be unaware. These are things happening on subtle levels, on tissue levels, on inner organ levels that may not having visible manifestations. Your body knows. Remember, nature is foolproof. When you start a healing and rejuvenation protocol, your body will send the nutrients to, or facilitate the cleansing of those systems and organs that need to be healed before other systems can be healed. Before healing your skin condition, for example, your body may need to heal your liver since the liver is a major organ of detoxification. Trust the body's innate intelligence to reverse the deterioration in the appropriate sequence. Discipline, patience and consistency are essential for true healing.

The instantaneous, overnight, magic pill type of healing that we've been led to expect from healing treatments is really just the suppression of symptoms. It is not real healing. Real healing, just like the real deterioration that took years of bad living to develop, may also take some time to reverse.

The good news, however, is that while it does take some time, it often does not take as many years to heal as it did to fall ill. I've heard some practitioners say it takes 1 month of healing for every 1 year of deterioration. I've heard others say it takes 2 weeks for every 1 year. It doesn't really matter who's correct, because everybody's body is different. The point is, you must respect the natural sequence and trust your body's intelligence.

Remember, nature's way is a slow single lane. This transitional period cannot be rushed. Most real cure cannot happen overnight. Part of the new paradigm involves respecting the intelligence of gradual cure at Nature's pace.

There is also an adjustment period as even your taste buds will need to adjust to the new tastes you are providing.

152. ❑ Expect: They will simply know! ❑

I'm going to suggest that once you start implementing the protocol, you'll be sending out different vibrations and energy. The people you wish to attract will know. Trust me! Call it the glow of health. Call it pheromone action. Call it whatever you like. Humans, like other animals, are drawn to partners who can complement their genes. Once you're radiating breeding vibrancy and not walking under a cloud of impotence, you might find your dating life miraculously improving!

153. ❏ The Process: Purge, prepare & plant ❏

The body in its toxic state is like a weed-filled garden, it requires you to first remove toxins (purge the weeds), then create the right environment for optimal assimilation of food (prepare the soil, then provide the best food (plant the best seeds) in order to create a garden of health. If any of these steps is missing, the whole plan breaks down. Think about it, if you ingest good food in a polluted system, you won't get maximum benefit. If you have a clean system but ingest garbage, it'll start to deteriorate. It's all about keeping the cells and tissues of the body clean. Here is more detail:

154. ❏ The Process: Purge ❏

Purging the body means taking any necessary steps to remove the accumulation of toxins, poisons, pills, drugs and waste that is in your system. For some, this may be a salt water wash and a fast, for some, a special sauna designed to sweat out toxins. For others a 14-day detox program that includes colonics, enemas, or special herbs like black walnut, oil of oregano, or grapefruit seed extract to kill parasites. It may be any combination of detoxes for the liver, kidneys, blood, and colon. It can be coffee enemas. The goal is to encourage the flow of bad stuff out of your system. You'll release the bad stuff in your stool, in your urine, in your perspiration or sloughed off your skin. I've done and still do all of these.

155. ❏ The Process: Prepare ❏

Once the soil in your garden is purged, you need to prepare it to be sure it can sustain the new growth. In our bodies, that equates to creating an environment that supports maximum absorption of nutrients. This may include enzymes to aid in digestion, it may include probiotics (eg. Acidophilus) to replenish the necessary intestinal flora in the colon.

156. ❏ The Process: Plant ❏

The final step in growing your garden would be to plant the best seeds to get the best crops. For us, this means replacing phony food with nutrient-rich, raw, live, natural, real food, taking whole food or liquid multivitamins, natural supplements, and eating high up on the Food Scale.

Purge, Prepare & Plant is not a one-time process. Even on a daily basis, everything I do, starting in the morning, is based on purging, preparing and planting my system. I start with lemon water in the morning to encourage an evacuation before I eat. If I eat breakfast that day, I'll usually always have raw fruit that has digestive enzymes, and/or start the day with a green juice and probiotic supplement.

157. ❏ Quick Start: Keep a daily log ❏

Keep a daily log of all that you do, what you experience, how often you have bowel movements, as well as the dreams, thoughts and ideas that come to you. There's a "30 Day Log" in Resources to help develop new habits.

158. ❏ Quick Start: Start Right NOW! ❏

DO TODAY…IMMEDIATELY…RIGHT NOW!!

☐ throw away white sugar, table salt, coffee

☐ place an order with an online vendor

☐ go shopping today or tomorrow at a health food store, and, if nothing else, get ground, organic coffee and distilled water and an enema kit or small enema bottles to do your first coffee enema

☐ join the Steel Pipe newsletter list at www.fittobreed.com

☐ Perform a one-day fast. Starting at a specific hour of the day, commit to doing nothing but drink water for a full 24 hours until that precise time the next day. Note: You will not die.

159. ☐ Quick Start: Do the blood work ☐

A single drop of blood from a pinprick, analyzed under a microscope and explained by an experienced naturopath can show you parasites (if you've got any), white blood cells, as well as the effects of poor diet and dehydration on the clustering and movement of your cells. Not critical, but would be a good "before" snapshot to compare later when you're fit to breed!

160. ☐ Quick Start: Initial phase ☐

Focus on remediation. Our goal during this initial phase is to flood the body with nutrients. Start Juicing. Start eating super foods. Start taking greens packs. Start drinking more water. We do this to provide the body and the immune system and repair system with necessary boost it will need to heal the body during the subsequent states. There will be some healing crises as your body starts to respond to this influx of nutrition, and even though your system may be polluted and even though your colon may not be in the best condition to absorb *all* the nutrients, there will still be benefit to providing your body what might be much-need vitamins, minerals. Let the healing begin!

161. ❏ Quick Start: Phase 2 ❏

Focus on purging. Continue the items in Phase 1. Experience your first salt water wash. Do you first fast. Perform a colonic. Do your first dry sauna. Eliminate late evening meals and have your heaviest meal during midday hours. You'll sill be eating during this phase, but you'll also be transitioning and incorporating elements of all

162. ❏ Quick Start: Phase 3 ❏

Focus on preparation of the intestinal system. Continue the items in Phases 1 & 2. Eat miso, kimchee, cultured vegetables and take probiotics as ways of restoring the good bacteria and intestinal flora.

163. ❏ Quick Start: Phase 4 ❏

Focus on real food and alkalinity. Continue the items in Phases 1, 2 & 3. Eat organic fruits and vegetables. Eat more alkaline-producing foods. Increase the amount of live, raw, sprouted, uncooked food in your daily diet. Eliminate canned, frozen or prepared foods from your diet.

Following are some recipes to help you put the protocol into action!

164. ❏ Quick Start: daily routine ❏

Here's a sample of a day in the life of the fit to breed.

6:000am   H202 on an empty stomach (see schedule)

6:00am   Lemon water in the morning

7:00am   Bowel movement

7:30am   Exercise on empty stomach

8:00am   Smoothie w/probiotic

9:00am   Breakfast:

Vitality Cereal, or Morning Reboot

12:00pm   Main meal between noon and 3pm:

option: Stir-fried veggies, Power cole slaw,

option: brown rice, Rock Hard salad, kimchee

3:00pm   Green Juice/CockTale snack dried fruit

5:00pm   Bowel movement

Notes:

no food in am until after first bowel movement
water throughout the day
coffee enemas in the evenings
no liquids with meals; 1.5 hours later

Fit to Breed Recipes for Two

Dishes to replenish and boost two people. Quantities are all flexible according to your taste and preferences.

Breakfast

165. ❑ Recipe: "ReVitalized" Cereal ❑
Cereal of choice (wheat/gluten-free; avoid corn)
rice/soy/almond milk   dash cinnamon
¼ cup bee pollen   1tbsp ground flax seeds
goji berries   ¼ cup raisins
raw pumpkin seeds   maca
Directions: sprinkle all ingredients onto cereal & milk

166. ❑ Recipe: "Morning After" Reboot Fruit ❑
A refreshing post play date breakfast!
med papaya   maca soy/coconut yogurt
1 mango   cinnamon
2 bananas   maple syrup
¼ c bee pollen   pineapple (sweetens of semen)
Directions: cube fruits, sprinkle with pollen, cinnamon, maca.

Lunch & Dinner

167. ❑ Recipe: "Endurance" Salad ❑
3 Cucumbers   1 tbsp kelp
3 Asparagus stalks   1 tbsp Irish moss
2tbsp moringa powder   1 tbps dulse
1-2oz olive oil   1 tbsp spirulina
Directions: Dice cucumbers and asparagus, Add garlic/ ginger/ cayenne/ salt. Mix together.

168. ❑ Recipe: "Constantleee" Coleslaw ❑
"If you were my woman, I would be making love to you

constantleee!" says the virile and well-endowed Dexter St. Jacques as he consoles a distraught tourist in Eddie Murphy's classic stand-up comedy sketch from the 1980s.

½ med. cabbage   ½c ground pumpkin seeds
1 carrot   1oz mustard   1oz apple cider vinegar
1tbsp spirulina   ½ avocado   garlic/ginger/cayenne/salt
Directions: Grate cabbage, carrots, mash in avocado. Mix all.

169. ❑ Recipe: Resurrection Soup (congee) ❑

Congee is a nutritive soup of grains cooked until dissolved, combined with healing herbs. The mixture is poured over live food that then becomes "cooked" by the heat of the soup. Congee dissolves fat, strengthens the kidneys and reverses the aging process. Buddha refers to congee as the food of longevity.

To prepare congee, you'll need: brown rice, teff, food herbs, millet, black beans (optional), dulse flakes, distilled or filtered water, and a crock pot. Pour ¼ cup of each grain (millet, rice, teff) into the pot. Add beans. Fill to brim with water, cover and cook on low overnight. Serve hot. Pour over greens. Season with dulse. Other types of ingredients may be added depending on the particular nutritive and curative results desired.

Juices & Smoothies

170. ❑ Recipe: "Infinite Duration" Juice ❑

4 celery stalks   spinach/ greens

2 carrots   grapefruit seed extract

3 apples   2 med bulbs ginger

Directions: Combine ingredients in juicer; take w/probiotics

171. ❑ Recipe: "ComeBack" CockTale ❑

This alone may be worth the price of admission! An original concoction I take daily that keeps me going strong!

12-16oz coconut water or apple juice
1-2 oz apple cider vinegar
1 tbsp maca
1 tbsp chlorophyll (100mg)
1 tbsp black seed oil
1 packet greens powder
1 packet electrolyte powder
3-5 drops grapefruit seed ext
1 oz trace mineral solution*
1oz DMSO
    Directions: combine all ingredients, close jar, and shake!
Open carefully. The electro-mix cause pressure buildup!
    The amounts are flexible. Use more or less of each as
you choose. May have a cleansing effect the first time.
**Some brands of trace minerals taste very salty. Sun Warrior
Liquid Light has a pleasant taste that won't overpower.*

172. ❑ Recipe: "Round Two" Smoothie ❑
8oz rice milk   ½ cup cashews
2 bananas   organic maple syrup to taste
1oz honey/molasses   ¼ cup pumpkin seeds
¼ cup bee pollen   ¼ cup Irish moss powder
maca   soy/coconut yogurt (optional)
Directions: combine in blender

Snacks

173. ❑ Recipe: "On the Comeback Trail" mix ❑
    raw cashews your favorite nuts pumpkin seeds
    raisins goji berries
Directions: Mix all together and start your comeback!

174. ❑ Recipe: "Power Your Stuff" cookies ❑
Stick to these amounts:
1/4 cup mix of organic almonds, organic whole flax seeds
1 cup gluten free oats   Pinch of cloves*

3 tbsp almonds*   2 tbsp maple butter
1 tbsp unsweet. coconut flakes 1/2 cup maple syrup
1tsp baking soda   3.5 tbsp coconut oil
1tsp baking powder 2 tsp vanilla
1/2 tsp cinnamon*   1/3 cup dates*
1/2 tsp sea salt   1/3 cup choc chips semisweet (opt)
1 tblsp raisins
Soak 1/4 cup oats in water for 15-30 min.
Place remainder of oats in a food processor
Do the same to the almond+flax+coconut flakes.
Combine all dry ingredients in a bowl.
Drain oats and add them to mix (save liquid)
Mix all wet ingredients in a small bowl; combing into dry and stir.
Add coconut flakes.
Chop almonds and the dates and add to mixture.
Add extra liquid if mix is stiff. Should not be too hard to scoop out
Slightly oil a baking pan with coconut oil
Use an ice cream scooper, scoop balls of mix onto baking sheet
Place in 350• oven for 12-15 min or until brown on top.
items can be adjusted to taste, replaced with others and possibly omitted depending on allergies and/or likes/dislikes.

175. ❑ Recipe: Cooking tips! ❑

Tip: Sprinkle nutritional yeast, spirulina, kelp, cayenne to any recipe to experiment while adding nutritive value to each dish!

Tip: don't overcook your meals. Stir fry for just a bit. Steam until still crunchy rather than boil until dead. Soak and sprout rather than cook. Raw, living food has more enzymes and is the way Nature intended them to be consumed.

Tip: I do not use many spices in my cooking, preferring a simple garlic/ginger/cayenne/salt combination for most meals.

Visit www.fittobreed.com for more recipes!

The Future ▲

For the purists!
Putting the "forever" in Fit to Breed

Here are some additional concepts and strategies to help you take the Fit to Breed lifestyle into the future and make it last forever!

176. ❑ Forever: Make the choice ❑

As you can see, the cures for all of these causes of impotence are in your hands. They are not the patented for profit "cures" offered by pharmaceutical companies. The *Fit to Breed* cures are all things you can do yourself for pennies, and some require only courage, discipline and the willingness to think and act little differently. The cures are straightforward and simple, but admittedly not easy in this society we live in.

Perhaps you were looking for an overnight cure. Perhaps you were looking for a pill you could take that could make everything all right. That is the unfortunate result of a lifetime of brainwashing by a medical industry that's all too happy to sell you products that purport to provide quick fixes, but which keep you tied to them for more "cures" for the further deterioration that comes as a result of the original cure.

Which brings us again to what this manual is all about--choice. Knowing what you now know about impotence, it's causes and cures, what choice will you make? Will you take the slower path back, or the quick fix?

My goal is not to chastise you or make you feel guilty for making either choice. You're an adult, free to make any choice you see fit. However, as I see it, you have two choices:

1. Keep doing what you're doing, and continue to droop, seeking temporary pharmaceutical remedies and little blue pills that come with a host of other side effects, or

2. Grow up and change your habits.

177. ❑ Forever: The discipline ❑

After a lifetime of excess, it is not habitual to eat one meal a day or to fast for an extended period. After a lifetime of immediate gratification, it is not habitual to practice disciplined delay. After a lifetime of eating anything that's placed in front of you, it is not habitual to be discriminating and selective.

178. ❑ Forever: The paradox of change ❑

There's no disputing that maintaining the Fit to Breed™ lifestyle is a challenge in modern times. There are distractions. There is false advertising. There are outright lies all designed to maintain the status quo. There is even your own personal resistance to what you are doing.

The ultimate paradox is that overcoming the depletion and toxicity of being unfit to breed requires discipline in order to change. However, those same conditions make it harder to exercise discipline, not just mentally, but physically as well. In other words, because your body may be suffering from certain deficiencies, and addictions, there are real biological cravings and withdrawal you may experience as you try to change.

The good news, however, is that human spirit and willpower are ultimately more powerful than any drugs. People have quit smoking, gotten themselves of addictive drugs and reversed lifetimes of bad habits purely by the exercise of will. Yes, change is possible. However, even if you have the willpower, there is still a further component to the paradox:

According to writer Sam Silverstein, people resist change because of a variety of reasons including:(a) Fear of change.(b)The uncertainty that change involves.(c)Trying new things is uncomfortable.(d) Difficulty with poor results until the benefits of change come.(e) People don't want to lose control. The paradox, therefore, is that *"Change is scary, but people only accept change when they feel safe."*

In a study involving 872 people who were specifically trying to change their *smoking* habits, psychologists Carlo DiClemente, Ph.D., and James Prochaska, Ph.D., identified five stages of change. These stages include:

precontemplation,
contemplation,
preparation,
action, and
maintenance.

I'll paraphrase their findings—extrapolating them to apply to our Fit to Breed journey:

"Once in the contemplation stage, people were most likely to respond to feedback and education as sources of information (eg. this book, *Fit to Breed*). Preparation stage folks were committed to changing and seeking a plan of action (eg. the Fit to Breed™ Protocol). Those in the action and maintenance stages were actively changing their behaviors and environments and found that social re-inforcers were important (eg. coaching, social network groups, online forums, support groups, etc.). Those who had relapsed were found to cycle back into earlier stages as they geared up to try again."

179. ❏ Warning: Brace for the attacks ❏

They will attack this. If this book gets too popular, people will attack it for a host of reasons including the references to various herbs, H2O2, DMSO, oil pulling, soul age, and other products, practices and beliefs. As author, my "credentials and qualifications" may be called into question. My character may be assassinated, all under the guise of protecting you, the consumer from harm. However, the real reason will be because *Fit to Breed* encourages you to bypass allopathic medicine, pharmaceutical companies and the medical establishment and cure yourself.

Don't worry, though. I'll survive any such attacks, and I'll continue to live my chosen lifestyle. However, the really unfortunate part of such smear campaigns (negative reviews, attacks on Amazon, claims of quackery on Wikipedia etc.) is that *you* and others who wish to heal yourselves, may start to doubt your ability to make informed, truth-based decisions about your health as your own authority.

Now, while it's true that some natural substances *can*, in fact, be harmful if overused or used incorrectly (no more so than the monosodium glutamate the Food and Drug Administration allows to be sold in stores, or the provably Alzheimer's-causing aluminum allowed in antiperspirants), 99% of what is advocated in *Fit to Breed* consist simply of proven plants and practices that have endured for thousands of years, spanned several continents and crossed many cultures in their use and effectiveness! These are truths and practices that have not changed in thousands of years, and did not require any outsider's approval to legitimize. They have been tested by history and culture. Their unfamiliarity to you—or to your well-meaning, but woefully nutritionally untrained doctor—is not reason to condemn or fear them. A doctor with the same degree and credentials, who happened to be Peruvian, would have an entirely different opinion about maca, would she not? (Just using maca as a random example to make a point.)

Don't let anyone tie you up in a meaningless debate and force you to defend or second-guess your chosen position and decisions. Remember what we said at the beginning of this journey: you don't need anyone's permission to eat an apple. You don't need anyone's approval to stop eating for a day. You don't need anyone's okay to feed your body in any way you wish to. Don't allow others' opinions to dissuade you. You don't need research to "prove" what you already know: apple=good; chemicals=bad.

As I said in the introduction, you are your own authority. Just as an example, maca is a root vegetable just like sweet potatoes. If you grew up in Peru, you'd be more familiar with it and likely be eating it every day. Don't let anyone convince you it's "untried" or "untested" or that "more studies are needed." There are a heckuva lot of healthy Peruvians. There are a lot of virile Jamaicans who drink Woodroot. There are a heckuva lot (a whole lot!) of Chinese who take ginseng! These cultures didn't need any outsider's endorsement, approval or permission to use them. So, even as you brace for any attacks, know that the power to become fit to breed is now—and has always been —in your hands!

I'll end this chapter with what the Ageless Adept think is one of the most profound statements in *The Man Who Lived Forever:*:

"Disappointed, Seeker? How much simpler and magical do you want it to be? You know, the most insane thing about our society is its insanity. The best definition I've heard for insanity is 'doing the same thing over and over and expecting different results.' We've been sold a childish belief that we can continue our destructive behavior, yet expect to reap creative benefits. We want to taste the sugar, but not its effects. We want to live in excess, without the accumulation. Then we place our hopes in magic pills or potions that we hope will wipe away the effects of our actions. But every truth in the universe supports an underlying order. That order is not a limitation. Quite the contrary, that order offers you unlimited potential. But at the same time, that order comes at a price, and cannot be violated.

"So, no, there is no super-food, magic pill, incantation, potion or magical fountain. But this, my friend, this is ten times better, because it is achievable; achievable by anyone who truly desires it. You are the magic itself. Your very being screams as proof of the magic of the universe. Your brain and its access to mind, your body and its access to life are all expressions of a magic that is your birthright from a magical universe. Within the Seven Conversations exists the phenomenal secret that you've come here to this planet already coded with the power of creation. But it is only through realignment with the truths of the universe and the truths of your being that you will ever be able to wield that magic power and create the results you desire.

"However, in your current state of brainwashing--in your delusion--you have missed the earth shattering significance of what you've just discovered. Here in your hands is the only workable approach to creating real magic that can exist in an ordered universe. You've just learned that you can, in fact, have perfect health, live longer and return to the days of your youth, and all you have to do is live according to natural law. You've just learned that every effect you desire is achievable given the right sequence of steps. And you miss the fact that it's the only approach that makes any sense. Any other approach would violate the laws of the universe. No, my friend, it doesn't get any more magical than it already is. Children seek magic on the outside. Adults find it within.

180. ❏ Forever: The Philosophy & Formula ❏

I hope you've gotten some benefit from *Fit to Breed*, the latest book in the Ageless Adept™ series. I'll end by sharing the underlying philosophy and formula for this series:

"If you can find the courage and discipline to eat only what exists in nature, avoid unnatural substances and environments, bask daily in sunshine, maintain direct contact with the earth, breathe clean air, purge the colon, cleanse the system, fast when dis-eased, and live passionately and on purpose from a belief system of universal perfection... you can prevent illness, reverse aging, rejuvenate the body, achieve perfect health and long life and become your own fountain of youth!"

My hope is that, just as I did, you and your partner(s) will do the work to change your beliefs, find the courage to embark on a new course of action, and find the discipline to sustain it until you are once again, reclassified as.....

FIT TO BREED.....forever!

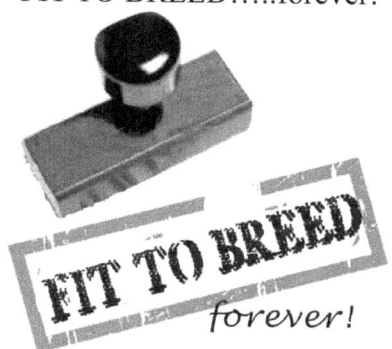

Walt F.J. Goodridge
The Fit to Breed Coach!

The Test ▲

What's your Fit to Breed Score?

181. ❑ Test: Take the Test ❑

This test accounts for past/present transgressions, environment, and beliefs to determine your Fit to Breed Quotient: the risk for impotence or compromised sexual function now or in the future.

1. Do you do coffee enemas?
a. No, never
b. In the past
c. Occasionally
d. Often

2. How many bowel movements do you have each day?
a. Less 1 (every 2+ days)
b. 1
c. 2
d. 3+

3. Do you seek out organic produce?
a. Not really
b. Seldom
c. Often
d. Religiously

4. How much <u>direct</u> sunlight do you get? (not through windows)
a. None, really
b. Less than an hour/day
c. More than an hour/day
d. I'm a sun worshipper!

5. How often do you exercise?
a. No time for it
b. Monthly
c. Weekly
d. Each day

6. How often do you eat at fast food restaurants?
a. Every day
b. once a week
c. once a month
d. Once a year to never

7. What about smoking?
a. I chain smoke
b. I smoke occasionally
c. Someone in my home does
d. Not I nor anyone at home

8. What about drinking/alcohol consumption?
a. I may have a problem
b. I drink occasionally
c. Someone in my home does
d. Not I nor anyone at home

9. Do you take any antibiotics?
a. In the past
b. Not sure/can't recall
c. Yes, currently
d. Never

10. Have you tested as a "Type A" personality?
a. Yes
b. Don't know
c. No

11. Complete: "GMO foods (genetically modified) are..."
a. safe to consume
b. the jury is still out; further testing is required.
c. harmful to the body and environment

12. Complete: "Direct exposure to the sun...."
a. runs the risk of causing skin cancer
b. the jury is still out; further scientific studies necessary
c. is helpful to the body's optimal function

13. Do you fast?
a. Never
b. In the past
c. Yes, perhaps once a year
d. Yes, more than once/year

14. Ever do colonics?
a. Never
b. In the past
c. Yes, perhaps once/year
d. Yes, more than once/year

15. What about your job/career?
a. I hate it with a passion!
b. It's just to pay the bills
c. I actually like what I do
d. Found my purpose/ passion!

Women: Do you take birth control pills or have an IUD?
a. In the past
b. yes currently
c. No. Never

Men: How often do you ejaculate? (masturbation+intercourse)
a. one or more times per day
b. once per week
c. once per month or less

❑ Test: How to score yourself ❑
Give yourself:

0 points for every "a" answer

1 point for every "b" answer

2 points for every "c" answer

3 points for very "d" answer

❑ The Test: What your score says!* ❑
Maximum score is: 45

☐ *Range: 0-11*

Your system is compromised. If smoking and alcohol are part of your profile, your score may even be tending into the negative range. It is likely you are already experiencing symptoms that indicate deeper underlying issues.

☐ *Range 12-23*

While still a better range to be in, your score indicates that there are some challenges. If not already manifesting, your sexual dysfunction is on its way sooner than later.

☐ *Range: 24-35*

Depending on your calendar age vs. biological age, this range shows you are more health-active (not just health conscious) than most, and may be aware of certain liberating beliefs that bode well for your future sexual health!

☐ *Range: 36-45*

You're a Fit to Breed all-star! Things can always be improved, but a score in this range shows you're doing all the right things to keep yourself and your partner(s) satisfied.

*This is only a sample of the full Fit to Breed Health Test. The online version, equipped with your calendar age, gender, lifestyle and beliefs, as well as the *specific* responses for each question, provides more details and recommendations. Take it online at http:/www.fittobreed.com

The Resources▲

Books, videos, websites & more

182. ❏ Food: Substitution shopping list ❏

AVOID: Milk, butter, eggs, cheese, chicken, all meats
processed sugar and salt, all foods with artificial flavor
preservatives & color of any kind, alcohol
cigarettes, sodas, fried foods, hybrid rice and wheat
products, processed white flour, decaffeinated coffee
All hybrid and genetically modified foods

ITEMS TO AVOID	REPLACE WITH
white sugar	maple syrup, honey, stevia
white rice	brown rice, millet, quinoa
white flour	rice flour, spelt flour, chick peas flour
milk	soy milk, almond or rice milk
soda	fresh-squeezed juices, water, herb teas
meat	curried eggplant, lentil, mushrooms
	stewed peas, soy beans, tofu, tempeh
	faux meat products
cheese	soy cheese or rice cheese
coffee, tea,	herb teas, green juice as pick-me-up
butter, margarine	olive oil, palm oil, pumpkin seed oil
table salt	sea salt, rock salt, Celtic salt
grain vinegar	apple cider vinegar, coconut vinegar
canned produce	fresh, organic produce
corn syrup, jam, jelly	nut butter
cooking oil	coconut oil

183. ❑ Food: Alkaline to Acid Food Chart❑

THE AGELESS FOOD SCALE : ALKALINE TO ACIDIC
The body's code is activated at a slightly alkaline pH of between 7.35–7.45 (Ideal 7.365)

EXTREMELY ALKALINE-FORMING
Lemons, watermelon, tangerine, and pineapple.
Baking soda, sea salt, mineral water, pumpkin seed, lentils, seaweed, onion, taro root, sea vegs, lotus root, swt potato, lime, lemons, nectarine, persimmon, raspberry,

ALKALINE-FORMING
Cantaloupe, cayenne, celery, dates, figs, kelp, limes, mango, melons, papaya, parsley, Asparagus, fruit juices, grapes (sweet), kiwifruit, passionfruit, pears (sweet), raisins, umeboshi plums, and vegetable juices.

MODERATELY ALKALINE-FORMING
Apples (sweet), alfalfa sprouts, apricots, avocados, bananas (ripe), currants, dates, figs (fresh), garlic, grapefruit, grapes (less sweet), guavas, herbs (leafy green), lettuce (leafy green), nectarine, peaches (sweet), pears (less sweet), peas (fresh, sweet), pumpkin, (sweet)

Apples (sour), beans (fresh, green), beets, bell peppers, broccoli, cabbage, carob, cauliflower, ginger (fresh), grapes (sour), lettuce (pale green), oranges, peaches (less sweet), peas (less sweet), potatoes (with skin), pumpkin (less sweet), raspberries, strawberries, squash, sweet Corn (fresh), turnip, vinegar (apple cider).

Apricots, spices, kambucha, unsulphured molasses, soy sauce cashews, chestnuts, pepper, kohlrabi, parsnip, garlic, asparagus, kale, parsley, endive, arugula, mustard green, ginger root, broccoli, grapefruit, cantaloupe, honeydew, citrus, olive, dewberry, carrots, loganberry, and mango.

Better

SLIGHTLY ALKALINE-FORMING

Almonds, artichokes (Jerusalem), brussel sprouts, cherries, coconut (fresh), cucumbers, eggplant, honey (raw), leeks, mushrooms, okra, olives (ripe), onions, pickles (homemade), radishes, sea salt, spices, tomatoes (sweet), vinegar (sweet brown rice), Chestnuts (dry, roasted), egg yolks (soft cooked), essene bread, goat's milk, whey (raw), mayonnaise (homemade), olive oil, sesame seeds (whole), soy beans (dry), soy cheese, soy milk, sprouted grains, tofu, tomatoes (less sweet), and yeast (nutritional flakes).

Most herbs, green tea, mu tea, rice syrup, apple cider vinegar, sake, quail eggs, primrose oil, sesame seed, cod liver oil, almonds, sprouts, potato, bell pepper, mushrooms, cauliflower, cabbage, rutabaga, ginseng, eggplant, pumpkin, collard green, pear, avocado, apples (sour), blackberry, cherry, peach, and papaya.

Better ↑

LOW ALKALINE-FORMING

Ginger tea, umeboshi vinegar, ghee, duck eggs, oats, grain coffee, quinoa, japonica rice, wild rice, avocado oil, most seeds, coconut oil, olive oil, flax oil, brussel sprout, beet, chive, cilantro, celery, okra, cucumber, turnip greens, squashes, lettuces, orange, banana, blueberry, raisin, currant, grape, and strawberry.

NEUTRAL ALKALINE-FORMING

Butter (fresh, unsalted), cream (fresh, raw), cow's milk and whey (raw), margarine, oils (except olive), and yogurt (plain).

VERY LOW ACID-FORMING
Curry, koma coffee, honey, maple syrup, vinegar, cream, butter, goat/sheep cheese, chicken, gelatin, organs, venison, fish, wild duck, triticale, millet, kasha, amaranth, brown ri rice, pumpkin seed oil, grape seed oil, sunflower oil, pine nuts, canola oil, spinach, fava beans, black-eyed peas, string beans, wax beans, zucchini, chutney, rhubarb, coconut, guava, dry fruit, figs, and dates.

LOW ACID-FORMING
Vanilla, alcohol, black tea, balsamic vinegar, cow milk, aged cheese, soy cheese, goat milk, game meat, lamb, mutton, boar, elk, shell fish, mollusks, goose, turkey, buckwheat, wheat, spelt, teff, kamut, farina, semolina, white rice, almond oil, sesame oil, safflower oil, tapioca, seitan, tofu, pinto beans, white beans, navy beans, red beans, aduki beans, lima beans, chard, plum, prune and tomatoes.

MODERATELY ACIDIC
Bananas (green), barley (rye), blueberries, bran, butter, cereals (unrefined), cheeses, crackers (unrefined rye, rice, and wheat), cranberries, dried beans (mung, adzuki, pinto kidney, garbanzo), dry coconut, egg whites, eggs whole (cooked hard), fructose, goat's milk (homogenized), honey (pasteurized), ketchup, maple syrup (unprocessed), milk

Molasses (unsulphured/organic), most nuts, mustard, oats (rye, organic), olives (pickled), pasta (whole grain), pastry (whole grain and honey), plums, popcorn (with salt and/or butter), potatoes, prunes, rice (basmati and brown), seeds (pumpkin, sunflower), soy sauce, wheat bread (sprouted org)

Nutmeg, coffee, casein, milk protein, cottage cheese, soy milk, pork, veal, bear, mussels, squid, chicken, maize, barley groats, corn, rye, oat bran, pistachio seeds, chestnut oil, lard, pecans, palm kernel oil, green peas, peanuts, snow peas, legumes, garbanzo beans, cranberry, pomegranate.

Better ↑

EXTREMELY ACIDIC-FORMING

Artificial sweeteners, beef, beer, breads, brown sugar, carbonated soft drinks, cereals, (refined), chocolate, cigarettes and tobacco, coffee, cream of wheat (unrefined), custard, (with white sugar), deer, drugs, fish, flour (white, wheat), fruit juices with sugar, jams, jellies, lamb.

Liquor, maple syrup (processed), molasses (sulphured), pasta (white), pastries and cakes, from white flour, pickles (commercial), pork, poultry, seafood, sugar (white), tablesalt (refined and iodized), tea (black), white bread, white vinegar (processed), whole wheat foods, wine, and yogurt (sweetened).

Brand name tabletop sweeteners pudding, jam, jelly, table salt (NaCl), beer, yeast, hops, malt, sugar, cocoa, white (acetic acid) vinegar, processed cheese, ice cream, beef, lobster, pheasant, barley, cottonseed oil, hazelnuts, walnuts, brazil nuts, fried foods, soybean, and soft drinks, especially cola type. To neutralize a glass of cola with a pH of 2.5, it would take 32 glasses of alkaline water with a pH of 10.

Better

184. ❏ Food: Superfood nutrient comparison ❏

Nutrient	Moringa	Bee Pollen	Spirulina	Chlorella
ENZYMES				
Disstase		✔		
Phosphatase		✔		
Amylase		✔		
Cataiase		✔		
Saccharase		✔		
Diaphorase		✔		
Pectase		✔		
Cozymase		✔		
Cytochrome		✔		
AMINO ACIDS				
Alanine	✔	✔	✔	✔
Arginine	✔	✔	✔	✔
Aspartic Acid	✔	✔	✔	
Cystine	✔	✔	✔	✔
Glutamic Acid	✔	✔	✔	
Glycine	✔	✔	✔	✔
Histidine	✔	✔	✔	✔
Isoleucine	✔	✔	✔	
Leucine	✔	✔	✔	✔
Lysine	✔	✔	✔	✔
Methionine	✔	✔	✔	✔
Phenylanaline	✔	✔	✔	✔
Proline	✔	✔	✔	✔
Threonine	✔	✔	✔	
Tryptophan	✔	✔	✔	✔
Tyrosine	✔	✔	✔	✔
Valine	✔	✔	✔	✔
Chlorophyll	✔		✔	✔
Protein	✔	✔	✔	✔
	Moringa	Bee Pollen	Spirulina	Chlorella

Nutrient	Moringa	Bee Pollen	Spirulina	Chlorella
Vitamin A (Beta Carotene)	✔	✔	✔	✔
Vitamin B1 (Thiamine)	✔	✔	✔	✔
Vitamin B2	✔	✔	✔	✔
Vitamin B3 (Niacin)	✔	✔	✔	✔
Vitamin B5 (Pantothenic Acid)		✔	✔	✔
Vitamin B6 (Pyridoxine)	✔	✔	✔	✔
Vitamin B12		✔	✔	✔
Vitamin C (Ascorbic Acid)	✔	✔	✔	✔
Vitamin D	✔	✔	✔	
Vitamin E	✔	✔	✔	✔
Vitamin H (biotin or Vit B7)	✔	✔		✔
Vitamin K	✔	✔	✔	
Choline			✔	
Folic Acid (B9)		✔	✔	✔
Rutin		✔		
Inositol		✔	✔	✔
Calcium	✔	✔	✔	✔
Phosphorous	✔	✔	✔	✔
Iron	✔	✔	✔	✔
Copper	✔	✔		✔
Potassium	✔	✔	✔	
Magnesium	✔	✔	✔	✔
Manganese	✔	✔	✔	
Silica		✔		
Sulphur	✔	✔		
Sodium	✔	✔	✔	
Iodine		✔		✔
Boron		✔		
Zinc	✔	✔	✔	✔
Selenium		✔	✔	
	Moringa	Bee Pollen	Spirulina	Chlorella

185. ❑ Hydrogen Peroxide cleansing schedule❑

Food grade hydrogen peroxide (H2O2) is available at health food stores and online in different concentrations. Take on an empty stomach, 1 hour before meals or 3 hours after. If taken too close to meals, it may react with bacteria in the food, causing foaming, indigestion and even vomiting. Avoid taking it too close to bedtime as it can energize you and result in sleeplessness. Here is a chart showing how many drops to use as a cleansing for the most popular concentrations.

Day #	Hydrogen Peroxide Concentration			Times Per Day
	3%	12%	35%	
1	20 drops	6 drops	2 drops	3
2	40 drops	12 drops	4 drops	3
3	60 drops	18 drops	6 drops	3
4	80 drops	24 drops	8 drops	3
5	100 drops	30 drops	10 drops	3
6	120 drops	36 drops	12 drops	3
7	140 drops	42 drops	14 drops	3
8	160 drops	48 drops	16 drops	3
9	180 drops	54 drops	18 drops	3
10	200 drops	60 drops	20 drops	3
11	200 drops	60 drops	20 drops	3
12	200 drops	60 drops	20 drops	3
13	200 drops	60 drops	20 drops	3
14	200 drops	60 drops	20 drops	3
15	200 drops	60 drops	20 drops	3
16	200 drops	60 drops	20 drops	3

Hydrogen peroxide is an extremely powerful cleanser for the blood and digestive tract. If your system is very toxic, you may experience a healing crisis. You may experience fatigue, diarrhea, headaches, skin eruptions, cold or flu-like symptoms, and nausea. If so, do not discontinue the hydrogen therapy. Simply go back to a lower number of drops and continue until the symptoms ease, then resume protocol.

186. ❏ Emotional Survival Scale ❏

Serenity		
Exhilaration		
Enthusiasm		
Cheerfulness		
Strong Interest		Surviving
Conservatism		
Mild interest		
Contentment		
Disinterest		
Boredom		
Antagonism		
Hostility		Succumbing
Pain		
Anger		
Hate		
Resentment		
No sympathy		
Unexpressed resentment		
Covert hostility		
Anxiety		
Fear		
Sympathy		
Grief		
Victim		
Hopeless		
Apathy		
Dying		
Death		

187. ❑ Books for more information ❑

❑ *Prescription for Nutritional Healing* by Phyllis & James Balch
This is a constant resource of natural remedies (vitamins, herbs, supplements etc.) for common ailments.

❑ *Arnold Ehret's MucusLess Diet & Healing System* by A. Ehret
Ehret explores the single underlying cause of all disease and explains it in lay language.

❑ *Rational Fasting* by Arnold Ehret
A sequel to Ehret's book

❑ *The Master Cleanser* by Stanley Burroughs
This little book contains the basis and instructions for the "lemonade fast" or "lemonade diet."

❑ *Diet For a New America* by John Robbins
John Robbins, son of the founder of Baskin & Robbins Ice Cream, exposed the horrendous and unsanitary conditions underlying the entire dairy and meat industries. One of the first books I read upon embarking on my journey.

❑ *Back to Eden* by Jethro Kloss
An amazing resource of herbs and natural remedies.

❑ *Why Do Vegetarians Eat Like That?* by David Gabbe
No longer in print, but still available online, this great introduction to vegetarianism is still one of my favorites!
❑ *Natural Cures They Don't Want You to Know* by Kevin Trudeau

An absolutely amazing expose, resource, guidebook and manual! You must own this and read Chapter 6 if nothing else!

☐ *Mad Cowboy* by Howard F. Lyman, Glen Merzer

☐ *Sugar Blues* by William Dufty

☐ *The Body Ecology Diet* by Donna Gates

☐ *Foods that Heal* by Bernard Jensen

☐ *How to Eat to Live* by Elijah Muhammad

☐ *Cleanse & Purify Thyself* by Richard Anderson

188. ❏ Books for improved sexual practices ❏

☐ *The Tao of Sexology*

☐ *Ancient Secret of the Fountain of Youth* by Peter Kelder
Originally published as *The Eye of Revelation.*

189. ❏ Books for Universal truth ❏

☐ The Kybalion *(in the public domain)*

190. ❏ Videos to change the world ❏

☐ The Gerson Miracle – cure for cancer and all disease

☐ The Beautiful Truth – cancer cure

☐ "Seeds of Death" and other award-winning documentaries
http://www.youtube.com/user/GaryNullTV

191. ☐ Websites for health information ☐

Research products and therapies, join communities of like-minded people, share and read testimonials.

☐ GaryNull.com – website of Gary Null

☐ Curezone.com

☐ Healyourselfathome.com

☐ Educate-yourself.org

☐ Shirleys-wellness-café.com

☐ EarthClinic.com

☐ NaturalNews.com - website of Health Ranger, Mike Adams

☐ Gerson.org – website of Charlotte Gerson's Gerson Therapy

192. ❏ Websites for purchasing products ❏

☐ Statmx.com – order Gerson Therapy products

☐ Vitaminlife.com – order just about everything else!

☐ Toolsforhealing.com – Zappers, organ cleanses.

☐ sota.com – colloidal silver maker, water ozonator

☐ discoveermms.com – MMS

☐ humaworm.com – Parasite cleanse

193. ❑ Fit to Breed Activity Log ❑

Copy and enlarge for your use.

The 30-Day Protocol Month: _____, Year: _____

Morning Item	1	2	3	4	5	6	7	8	9	10	11	12	13	14	15	16	17	18	19	20	21	22	23	24	25	26	27	28	29	30	31

Midday Item	1	2	3	4	5	6	7	8	9	10	11	12	13	14	15	16	17	18	19	20	21	22	23	24	25	26	27	28	29	30	31

Evening Item	1	2	3	4	5	6	7	8	9	10	11	12	13	14	15	16	17	18	19	20	21	22	23	24	25	26	27	28	29	30	31

194. ❑ FAQ to Breed ❑
Topics covered in the Ageless Living™ series

❑ What else do we lose that should be replenished?
SWEAT, *because it contains: Vitamin C, the B Vitamins Thiamine and Riboflavin, Lactate, Urea, Ammonia, Creatine, Uric acid, Chloride, Glucose,* and:
URINE contains: *Alanine, Arginine, Ascorbic acid Allantoin, Amino acids, Bicarbonate, Biotin, Calcium, Creatine, Cystine, Dopamine, Epinephrine, Folic acid, Glucose, Glutamic acid, Glycine, Inositol, Iodine, Iron, Lysine, Magnesium, Manganese, Methionine, Nitrogen, Ornithine, Pantothenic acid, Phenylalanine, Phosphorus, Potassium, Proteins, Riboflavin, Tryptophan, Tyrosine, Urea, Vitamin B6, Vitamin B12, Zinc.*
While some of the urine contains excess that the body doesn't use, some of it is also vitamins and mineral that are not adequately absorbed by the body—just another reason to focus on replenishment as a directive of the protocol.

❑ What are The Seven Conversations?
The Seven Conversations are the fascinating discussions "the man" has with "the seeker" in *The Man Who Lived Forever.* While the book's story is "somewhat fictional," the principles of health and longevity that form its foundation are real and form the basis of the very achievable, real-life Yesterday's You™ & Fit to Breed™ protocols: 1.Nature is foolproof. 2.The body is coded to heal. 3.There is only one disease. 4.There is only one cure. 5.Food and fasting facilitate flow. 6.There is one hindrance to health. 7.There is one challenge to change. And, there is a vital 8th conversation: 8.Every prior condition is achievable. The goal of these Seven Conversations (plus one) is to restore the seeker's certainty in his or her own viewpoint, her own perceptions, intuition and the ability to extrapolate the unknown from the known.

❑ What is Mucoid Plaque?

Answer by the man who coined the term, Richard Anderson, N.D., N.M.D., author of *Cleanse and Purify Thyself*: "The intestines can store a vast amount of partially digested, putrefying matter (as well as drugs and other toxic chemicals)—for decades even. Some intestines, when autopsied, have weighed up to 40 pounds and were distended to a diameter of 12 inches with only a pencil-thin channel through which the feces could move. That 40 pounds was due to caked layers of encrusted mucus mixed with fecal matter, bizarrely resembling hardened blackish-green truck tire rubber or an old piece of dried rawhide. I call this mucoid plaque. This mucoid plaque, when it is removed during an intensive colon cleanse, often shows ropelike twists, striations, overlaps, folds, creases—the shape and texture of the intestinal wall. Mucoid plaque may vary considerably, depending on the chemical conditions in a person's intestines. It may be hard and brittle; it may be firm and thick; tough, wet, and rubbery; soft, thick, and mucoid; or soft, transparent, and thin; it can range in color from light brown, black, or greenish-black to yellow or grey, and sometimes emits an intensely foul odor. I coined the term mucoid plaque, meaning a film of mucus, to describe the unhealthy accumulation of abnormal mucous matter on the walls of the intestines."

You absolutely cannot be fit to breed if you've got an accumulation of mucoid plaque in your colon!

☐ What are "Bitters?"

Bitter, salty, sweet and sour tastes all have important effects on the body. "Bitters," the roots, leaves of specific bitter-tasting herbs, are a time-honored, "old fashioned" remedy used in many cultures to rejuvenate vital organs, improve regularity, aid digestion, balance the system and rid the body of stomach disorders, worms, intestinal parasites, aiding liver function and much more...(Jamaican, Swedish, African, et.al.)

☐ If I fast for 10+ days, I'll starve!

The difference between fasting and starvation is

summed up by Hereward Carrington in *Fast & Grow Young*: "Fasting is a scientific method of ridding the system of diseased tissue, and morbid matter, and is invariably accompanied by beneficial results. Starving is the deprivation of the tissues from nutriment which they require, and is invariably accompanied by disastrous consequences. The whole secret is this: fasting commences with the omission of the first meal and ends with the return of natural hunger, while starvation only begins with the return of natural hunger and terminates in death. Where the one ends the other begins. Whereas the latter process wastes the healthy tissues, emaciates the body, and depletes the vitality; the former process merely expels corrupt matter and useless fatty tissue, thereby elevating the energy, and eventually restoring the organism that just balance we term health."

☐ Let the Hunger Names Begin! ☐

Hollow Hunger is the feeling of an empty stomach identifiable by rumbling/gurgling. I call it hollow also because this hunger disappears after the initial 1-3 days of a fast.

Habit Hunger is the longing for food—what some people call "mouth hunger" that just feels like you want to put something in your mouth and experience the sensation of chewing and swallowing. This is the habit of eating that is more in the mind and mouth than anywhere else.

Healing (Help!) Hunger happens on a chemical, system-wide level as your body really begins to call out for help and sustenance after the completion of the healing fast, the exhausting of your body's reserves, and the need to start replenishing certain nutrients for survival.

Fast & Grow Young teaches when it's time to give in to healing hunger. As you go through the Fit to Breed protocol (whether you fast or not), you'll get better at answering: "Am I really hungry, or is it just that time of day I habitually eat?" and discern between these different hunger names.

☐ What is Aging by Agreement?

I believe a lot of aging is simply the result of subtle,

subliminal, conscious and unconscious agreements we make every day to conform to society's concept of health, sickness, aging and death. *"Oh, you're just getting old."* *"That's what happens when you get to be our age."* These thoughts and words we agree with are not without effect. Purge these thoughts from your mind. Don't buy into them during conversations. Don't tell people your age. (Their thoughts about what that age "means" to them will get projected onto you.) Respond aloud if not just in your mind with: *"That may be true for you, but I'm getting younger every day!"* Dare to disagree.

☐ **Do you follow your own advice?**

Just about! I've acknowledged the existence of the first time failure and even talk about it with my lovers; I've accepted and pursued the type of women and attributes I like (pretty feet turn me on!); I've done the nomad thing in order to place and position myself in cultures in which and with which I feel a special alignment and synergy; I've embraced my dominant side; I've sought fulfillment by following my passion, and I've defined for myself what it means to be a man and to consider myself success at living. by taking care of my body, keeping it clean, toxin-free, and supplied with the necessary nutrients every single day. Read *"If you want to be my girlfriend..."* for more, even if you don't want to be my girlfriend!

☐ **The Protocol...That's a lot to do isn't it?**

First, I only recommend things I've personally tried and can vouch for. Second, remember that some of the products and processes I share were discovered at various stages of my own journey. For example, when it comes to cleanses, It was four years after becoming vegan that I discovered the Master Cleanser and did my first 10-day lemonade fast. Ten years later, I discovered colonics and coffee enemas. In between, I've done zapping, and the multi-day cleanses. So, even though they are all presented in a single protocol here, they are not all things you need to be doing all at one time, all the time. Start with a fast and coffee enema. Start with a few supplements and allow each one a few days/weeks to start to have an effect. Take your time. Don't rush. Don't overdo it or do everything at once.

However, if I had to choose five things to do within the first few days/weeks of the protocol, I would recommend: (1) doing a coffee enema, (2) adding the "Comeback CockTale" as a regular part of your day (3) doing some sort of colonic cleanse/irrigation (saltwater wash, colonic, multi-day cleanse), (4) fasting for at least 24 hours as an initial test of your discipline, and (5) some form of exercise.

☐ What are you not telling us?

In other words, what have you forgotten to mention that has really helped you remain fit to breed?

I've thought about this a lot and believe some of the subtle contributing factors to my overall health include:

(a) I started early. I became vegan about 5 years out of college. There was less deterioration to reverse.

(b) I quit my job. I no longer have that tremendous stress and unhappiness hovering over me.

☐ What is the salt water wash?

A harmless but thorough colon cleanse. Add 2 level tablespoons of non-iodized sea salt to 32 oz of water and stir over low flame until dissolves and lukewarm. Drink all early in the morning as quickly as you can. Mixture has the same specific gravity as blood, and is not absorbed by the colon. Washes through the system in anywhere from 2-4 hours; suggested as the first step before the lemonade fast.

☐ Why do I need probiotics/Acidophilus?

If you've ever taken birth-control pills or antibiotics, you'll need to consider restoring your body's balance of intestinal flora with probiotics. The imbalance they cause (often leading to Candida Albicans yeast overgrowth) is cited in a host of discomforts including chronic fatigue, loss of interest in intimacy, brain fog and more. Acidophilus is friendly bacteria which aids digestion, enhances immunity, alleviates allergies, fights yeast infections and more.

□ What are enzymes?

Enzymes are essential for life. Naturally-occurring in real food, they aid digestion, build proteins, carbohydrates and fats. Raw food has more enzymes than cooked food. A digestive enzyme supplement can enhance effectiveness of the digestive tract.

□ What's the body's vitamin/mineral composition?

96.2% of the body's weight is water, Carbon Dioxide, DNA, RNA proteins, lipids and sugars composed primarily of Oxygen (65.0%), Carbon (18.5%), Hydrogen (9.5%),Nitrogen (3.2%); The remainder is various salts comprised of Calcium (1.5%), Phosphorus (1.0%), Potassium (0.4%), Sulphur (0.3%),Sodium (0.2%), Chlorine (0.2%), Magnesium (0.1%), Iodine (0.1%), Iron (0.1%); Trace amounts (less than 0.5% of total body weight) of Chromium, Cobalt, Copper, Fluorine, Manganese, Molybdenum, Selenium, Tin, Vanadium and Zinc. These must be replenished for the body to retain youth, elasticity, immunity, vitality, energy, regenerative capacity, and structure over time. Science doesn't know everything required for the body's function. There are compounds, solutions, molecules (i.e. combinations of individual elements), in specific amounts affected by interaction with others, under specific conditions, which Nature has not divulged. Therefore, obtaining your nutrition for replenishment is best done by eating real foods and living as naturally possible.

195. ❑ Fit to Breed Test online ❑
☐ Health TEST: What's My Fit to Breed SCORE?

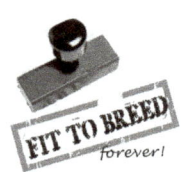

What's your Fit to Breed™ score? How has your lifestyle affected your FTB quotient? How do you compare with others who've taken the test? Answer a few questions, click "submit," and find out! *Take the latest version of the Fit to Breed™ online health test at www.fittobreed.com*

196. ❑ YOUR GOAL SETTING MANTRA ❑

One of the best and proven ways to achieve anything in life is to write it down repeatedly (with pen and paper) as a goal, in the present tense, with a deadline, every day upon waking. Here is a suggestion of how to write a "Fit to Breed" goal every day:

"I am fit to breed. My body is clean and free of all worms, parasites, viruses, bacteria, as well as organic, pharmaceutical and industrial toxins. My muscles are strong, my stomach is flat, my skin is clear and blemish-free, my libido is high and my ejaculate shoots out three feet or more all by [date]."

☐ Questions?

Email protocol questions to questions@agelessadept.com or visit www.agelessadept.com and post a comment to the blog.

197. ❑ Get to know the Ageless Adept ❑

"Perfect health, long life and eternal youth are not the random, genetic blessings of a chaotic or capricious universe, but natural birthrights that can be accessed through the mindful acceptance of simple truths, activated by the disciplined practice of proven protocols, and sustained by advancement along a known path. This is that path."

My name is Walt F.J. Goodridge, author and publisher of the *Ageless Adept™* series of books, and I'm here to prove a point!

Years ago, before I became vegan, a friend asked a question over lunch I couldn't answer. He asked, *"Do you know what's in the food you're eating?"* I did not, and as a trained engineer, it bothered me that I had failed such a simple test, and so--with health, longevity and vitality as my goals--I dedicated my life to a search for answers and ultimately to *"share what I know, so that others may grow."*

My childhood in the Caribbean steeped in me an understanding of and reverence for our natural world of sunshine, water, earth, air and time. As an adult, I discovered that what passes as *normal* health and healing in the western paradigm is shockingly *unnatural*! It never made sense to me that natural beings should need to turn to men in lab coats with pills in search of wellness. It makes more sense that Nature would have the answers built in; that our bodies would have an innate healing code; that our "operations manual" is simple and foolproof.

Through my own experiments, the testimonials of others of like mind, and the corroboration of researchers from this and previous eras, I've realized that the symptoms we as a society accept as a "normal" part of aging are simply the body's reactions to unnatural habits of ingesting pharmaceuticals, fake food with non-food ingredients, pesticides, hormones, steroids and antibiotics, as well as other environmental factors. Some of the causes (i.e. habits) may be hard to break, but are ultimately under our control and controllable. And, if the *causes* are controllable, then the *effects* are not inevitable and may even be reversible! That's what I'm here to prove!

I've distilled the results of my experiments into my Ageless Adept™ philosophy and protocols--information I hope will (1) empower you to become your own authority in matters of health, and (2) make better survival decisions choosing from among the products and practices you'll encounter on your own path of perfect health, long life and the fountain of youth!

198. ❏ Get to know the Ageless Adept Series ❏

Free books are available only from me:
www.agelessadept.com/shop

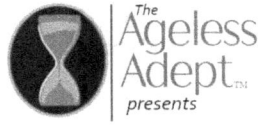

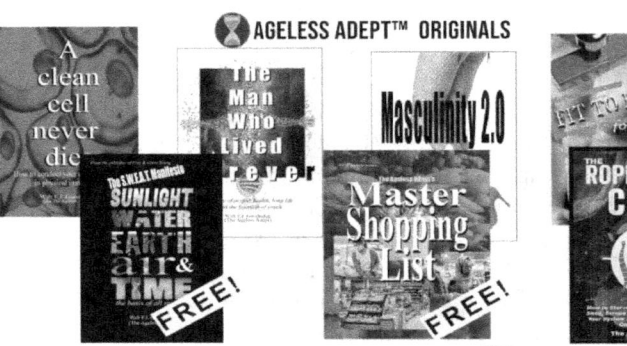

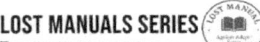

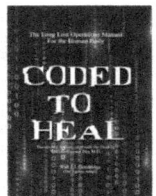
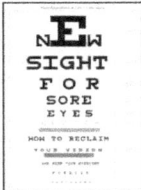
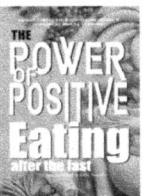
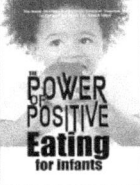
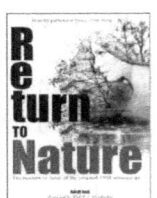

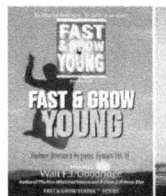
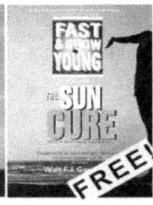
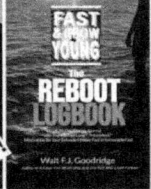
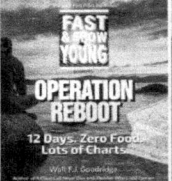
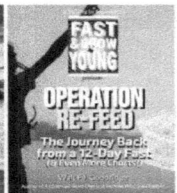

See also: www.fastandgrowyoung.com

199. ❑ Get Even More Free Stuff ❑

The Ageless Adept™ presents

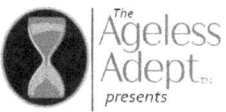

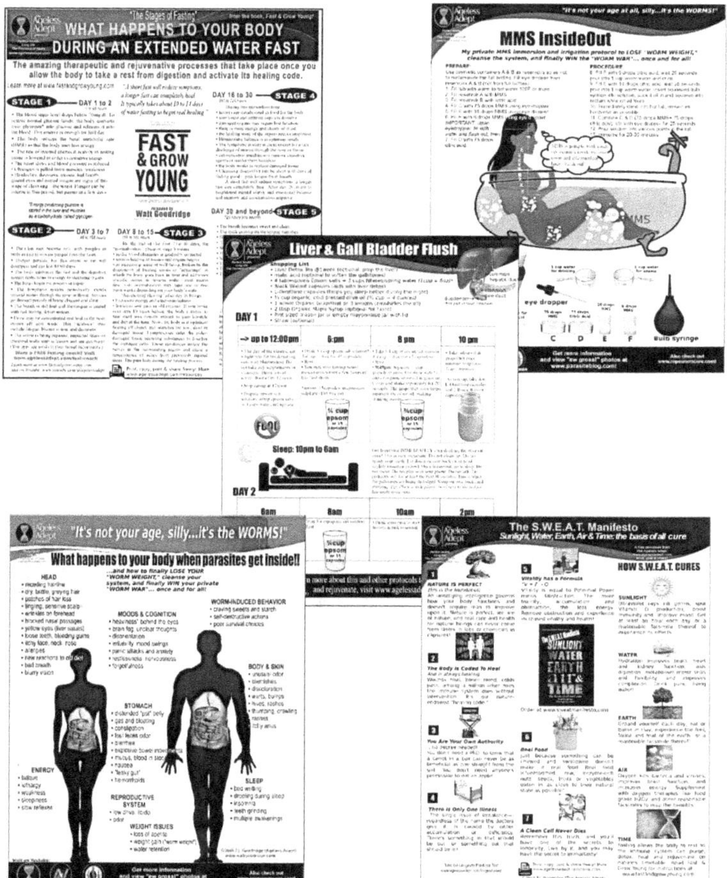

Book summaries, infographics, posters, charts with information and instructions for fasting, detoxing, parasite elimination and ageless living are available at www.agelessadept.com/downloads

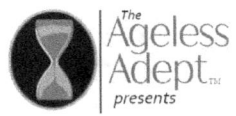

Youtube™ Channels

  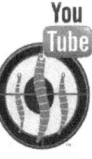

@agelessadept
@askavegan
@ropewormcure

Blogs

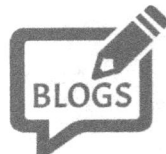

agelessadept.com/blog
parasiteblog.com

***

Merchandise

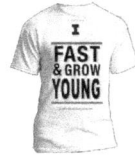 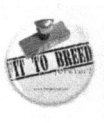

T-shirts, mugs, buttons and more!

Tests & Quizzes

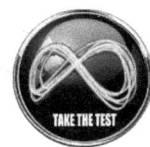 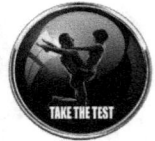

Longevity Test
Fit to Breed? Test

Available at www.agelessadept.com

Join the Ageless Adept Movement

"Get exclusive healing protocols, behind-the-scenes insight, and subscriber discounts on books & coaching."

https://www.agelessadept.com/newsletter

The Power of the Paperback ▲

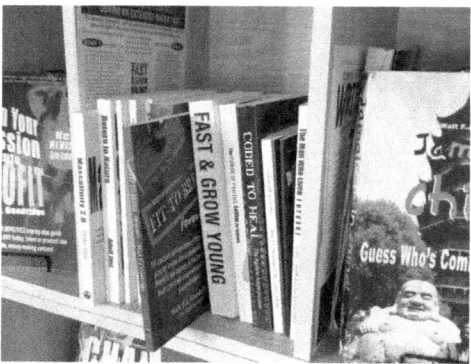

Digital books are convenient—but they're invisible, intangible, and easily forgotten. A paperback, on the other hand, has **mass, presence, and power**. It sits on your shelf, catches your eye, calls you back in, and keeps transmitting its wisdom long after you've turned the final page.

It whispers reminders, sparks curiosity in guests, and is far easier to share, gift, or revisit than a digital file lost in the cloud.

The paperback endures.

"Fit to breed" is more than just a title. It is a reminder as well as an optimistic ideal shared each time you or others glance at your shelf!

Order *https://www.agelessadept.com/shop*

***

Other Brands by the Author ▲

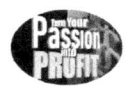 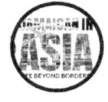 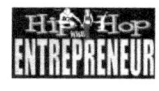 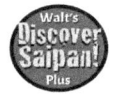

PassionProfit.com   JamaicaninAsia.com   HipHopEntrepreneur.com   DiscoverSaipan.com

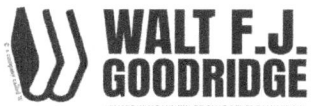

Or find them all at https://www.waltgoodridge.com